About This Book

If you've ever looked for a better way, a wiser way, a more fundamental way to improve your health, look no further. Here age-old principles of health and healing from the Maharishi Ayur-Veda tradition are described in clear, simple prose.

As the authors explain, there is an inner intelligence within each of us that governs and coordinates all the life processes of the body. "This is the same natural intelligence that orchestrates and coordinates the entire universe, . . . keeps the planets moving in their orbits, makes the seasons come on time, and prevents an apple or a peach from growing on a pear tree." The secret of staying forever healthy is simply to enliven this natural inner intelligence.

Maharishi Ayur-Veda knowledge is not new. This book tells where it came from, how it has been brought to light by Maharishi Mahesh Yogi, and why it can make a difference in your daily life.

Dr. Reddy speaks from experience—her own personal experience and the experience of her patients. Included are real case histories showing the power of the Maharishi Ayur-Veda approach, practical knowledge for you to apply in your own life right now, a summary of scientific studies that have validated this approach, and a complete chapter on where to go for more information in your local area.

All diseases do not need drugs. All patients with the same disease do not need the same treatment. Chronic disorders need not be chronic. Our health and quality of life do not have to deteriorate as we grow older. These are just myths that we have grown up with and often accept without question.

But more and more people are beginning to ask the question: What more can I do for my health? If you are one of them, you will find here real and helpful answers. From the oldest tradition in the world comes complete and time-tested knowledge to help you create an ideal state of health and well-being.

Maharishi Ayur-Veda health care is the ultimate holistic approach which treats every level of life—spiritual, mental, emotional, physical, behavioral, and environmental. Here is the concise introduction we have all been waiting for!

"An excellent introduction to Maharishi Ayur-Veda health care, for the physician and for the lay person. The principles of the Maharishi Ayur-Veda approach are explained thoroughly in clear, simple, delightful language that makes the book enjoyable to read and easy to understand. . . . This approach is very valuable for those in leadership positions, both in business and in government, because it is easily incorporated into existing systems of health care and offers tremendous practical benefits for the health of society as a whole."

Kurleigh King, Ph.D.
Director-General, Institute of World Leadership
Maharishi University of Management, Fairfield, Iowa
Secretary-General, Caribbean Community and Common Market
(CARICOM), 1978–1983

"This book represents the personal journey of a practicing medical specialist who desired increased ability to alter her patients' outcomes. . . . In no case should it be ignored by any individual who wishes to explore alternative medical therapies."

Philip D. Lumb, M.B., B.S., F.C.C.M.
Anesthesiologist-in-Chief, Albany Medical Center Hospital
Professor of Anesthesiology and Surgery
Chairman, Department of Anesthesiology
Albany Medical College, Albany, New York

FOREVER HEALTHY

Introduction to
Maharishi Ayur-Veda
Health Care

Preventing and Treating Disease through
Timeless Natural Medicine

by Kumuda Reddy, M.D. and Stan Kendz

Samhita Enterprises, Incorporated
Rochester, New York

Samhita Enterprises, Inc.
183 Saint Paul Street
Rochester, New York 14604
1-800-784-2773

®Maharishi Ayur-Veda, Maharishi Transcendental Meditation, Transcendental Meditation, TM, TM-Sidhi, Maharishi Vedic Approach to Health, Maharishi Rejuvenation, Maharishi Gandharva Veda, Gandharva Veda Music, Maharishi Sthapatya Veda, Maharishi Jyotish, Maharishi Yagya, Maharishi Yoga, Maharishi University of Management, Maharishi International University, Maharishi Vedic University, Maharishi Ayur-Veda University, Maharishi Vedic School, Maharishi Ayur-Veda School, Maharishi College of Vedic Medicine, Maharishi Ayur-Veda Medical Center, Maharishi Vedic Center, Maharishi Vedic Medical Center and Maharishi Amrit Kalash are registered or common law trademarks licensed to Maharishi Vedic Education Development Corporation and used with permission.

ISBN 1-57582-021-8

We gratefully acknowledge permission to use material from the following published sources. The charts and text on pages 142–147, 150–153, 156–163, and 170–175 are adapted from *Scientific Research on the **Maharishi Transcendental Meditation** and **TM-Sidhi** Programs: A Brief Summary of 500 Studies* (Fairfield, IA: Maharishi University of Management Press), © 1996 by Maharishi University of Management, and from *Scientific Research on the Maharishi Technology of the Unified Field: The **Transcendental Meditation** and **TM-Sidhi** Program* (Fairfield, IA: Maharishi International University Press), © 1988 by Maharishi International University. The charts and text on pages 148–149, 154–155, and 164–166 are adapted from *Maharishi Mahesh Yogi's **Transcendental Meditation*** by Robert Roth (New York: Donald I. Fine), © 1994 by WPEC–U.S. The chart on page 167 is adapted with permission from *Nutrition Research*, vol. 12, authors V.K. Patel, J. Wang, R.N. Shen, H.M. Sharma, and Z. Brahmi, "Reduction of Metastases of Lewis Lung Carcinoma by an Ayurvedic Food Supplement [MAK–4] in Mice," pp. 51–61, 1992, Elsevier Science Inc. The information presented in the chart and text on page 168 is taken from *Pharmacologist*, vol. 3, 1991, p. 39 (Abstract), with permission of the author, Brian Johnston. The chart and text on pages 176–177 is adapted from *Summary of Research Findings*, (Colorado Springs, CO: Maharishi Ayur-Veda Products International, Inc.), 1996. The illustration and caption on page 43 and the chart and caption on page 45 are adapted from *The Total Health Catalog*, vol. 2, 1994–1995, p. 7 and vol. 3, no. 1, Fall 1995, p. 18, © 1994 and 1995 by Maharishi Ayur-Veda Products International, Inc., Colorado Springs, Colorado.

To Maharishi Mahesh Yogi for giving us the vision to be forever healthy.

"Taking recourse to Maharishi Ayur-Veda means putting ourselves on the path of long life, the path of perfect health."   Maharishi Mahesh Yogi

Contents

Acknowledgments

We would like to give special thanks to Tony Nader, M.D., Ph.D. and Keith Wallace, Ph.D. for their encouragement and support, Richard Averbach, M.D. and Stuart Rothenberg, M.D. for their editorial review, Hema Reddy, M.D., Mike Tompkins, James Collins, Michael Moore, Laura Wysong, Susan Shatkin, Bill Groetzinger and the many others who supported this project. Most of all, we thank our families for their patience, understanding and love.

Preface

You might wonder how this book got started. Here is my story—how I discovered Maharishi Ayur-Veda® health care and why I felt inspired to share it with you by writing this book.

As a physician, I have had over 20 years of experience practicing conventional Western medicine. Because my specialty is anesthesiology, I always worked with serious and complicated cases in hospital settings. For many years my typical work-week was 60–70 hours long, most of it spent in operating rooms.

During all those years, it was an enormous concern in my mind and heart to find the cause of disease, to understand why patients were always going from doctor to doctor, and never finding lasting relief. It was this thought that led me to search for something more than conventional medicine—and yet something that would be complementary to conventional medicine as well.

It has been my experience that patients who are diagnosed and treated on the level of symptoms get better only to develop a new set of symptoms. There are many patients who even accept this cycle as a necessary part of life. Moreover, patients who have surgery often think that going from one operation to the next is a normal experience. They think that it is quite acceptable to have two or more surgeries in one's lifetime.

I refused to accept this definition of "normal." I began searching for a solution to the many problems experienced by my various patients. My search ended with the discovery of the Maharishi Ayur-Veda approach to health care several years ago.

Although I had heard about Ayur-Veda from my childhood in India, the wholeness of the knowledge was missing until its recent revival by Maharishi Mahesh Yogi. Historically, Ayur-Veda is the oldest form of natural holistic medicine, and elements of it are found in many other systems of health care.

Mankind has always been searching for health and happiness; one does not exist without the other. The Maharishi Ayur-Veda approach has helped me enormously, both personally and as a physician, to understand and experience well-being. Because I have experienced health and happiness myself through this comprehensive system of health care, it has been easy to incorporate the Maharishi Ayur-Veda approach into my practice and deliver that health care to everyone I meet.

In my practice, I have found that patients who try Maharishi Ayur-Veda therapies learn from their own experience that they have chosen the best and most complete form of natural medicine. Patients who still rely on conventional medicine but try Maharishi Ayur-Veda health care for that "something more" to bring additional health and vitality discover that it is extremely complementary. The simplicity, compatibility and efficacy of this system prove that it is ideal for everyone. It treats illness, creates health, and also helps us develop our full potential as human beings so that life becomes a glorious existence of joy and fulfillment.

Furthermore, knowledge from the Maharishi Ayur-Veda tradition addresses not just ourselves and our individual health, but the extension of ourselves—the universe itself, and the health of the entire universe. I believe that by beginning to understand this enormous, profound and truly compassionate knowledge we can become the creators of our own ideal health and also the means for creating a disease-free society.

What my co-author and I present in this book is basic knowledge about the Maharishi Ayur-Veda program, which will help you appreciate its benefits and show you where to go for more information. It is possible to spend many years studying this vast and rich field of knowledge; in this book we hope to give you a sampling of what is available. One can always learn more, but for knowledge to be real and useful it must be experienced for oneself. The Maharishi Ayur-Veda program is practical, and easy to apply to one's life. It is my profound desire that people of all ages, all races, all religions, all nationalities and all cultures use this universal knowledge for their own personal benefit and enjoy good health forever. Now is the best time to begin!

Kumuda Reddy, M.D.

Preface

I add my voice to that of Dr. Reddy's to mention my personal experience with the Maharishi Ayur-Veda program.

I was born and raised in New York City and lived what might be called an "average life." I was introduced to the Maharishi Ayur-Veda approach to health care in my mid-twenties, and over the years gradually incorporated various aspects of this timeless knowledge into my daily routine. I found that each time I added something new I enjoyed better health, more creativity, and a growing experience of inner joy and harmony. I also began to notice that my relationship with my environment was more fulfilling. My career became more satisfying and I became actively involved in community service. To my amazement and delight I began to enjoy a state of uninterrupted health more than a decade ago.

So from personal experience I know that disease can be prevented, and that one can live in harmony with one's environment.

Contributing to this book has been deeply fulfilling for me because it satisfies my desire to share the knowledge of Maharishi Ayur-Veda health care with others like myself. I consider myself to be an "average person" and I wanted everyone to know that it works for people like me. Everyone can enjoy the benefits of health and happiness just by making simple changes in their daily lives.

It is my hope that this book will motivate you to begin using this timeless system of total health care, so that you too can begin to experience the joys of living in freedom—particularly freedom from disease.

Stan Kendz

Part I

An Introduction to *Maharishi Ayur-Veda* Health Care

Part I will orient you to the Maharishi Ayur-Veda system of natural health care. In chapter one we define this system, tell you where it came from, and describe the key role that Maharishi Mahesh Yogi has played in making it available. We also briefly describe its various therapies (there will be more on Maharishi Ayur-Veda therapies in Part II), and review the growth of this system over the past ten years.

In the next few chapters, we discuss the advantages of using this unique system of health care. In chapter two we describe how Maharishi Ayur-Veda^{SM} knowledge brings a new vision of possibilities to health care. In chapter three we discuss how Maharishi Ayur-Veda therapies go beyond the surface level of symptoms. In chapter four, we discuss how the various Maharishi Ayur-Veda approaches are **safe** because they work holistically, **simple** because they are natural and work with the body's own inner intelligence, and **effective** because they operate on deeper, more powerful levels of the mind and body. In chapter five, we describe how the Maharishi Ayur-Veda system offers complete health care. It offers not only treatment for disease, but programs for prevention and rejuvenation as well. In chapter six, we compare Maharishi Ayur-Veda health care with conventional medicine, and discover that it works very well with the conventional approach. Moreover, it supplies what has been missing in conventional medicine and other healing technologies—effective strategies for preventing disease and creating perfect health in the individual and society as a whole.

A special advantage of the Maharishi Ayur-Veda approach is its ability to eliminate the root causes of disease. In chapter seven, we describe what causes disease, according to this age-old system of natural health care.

With this introduction to Maharishi Ayur-Veda health care in Part I, we will then go on in Part II to describe specific therapies for the prevention and cure of disease.

Chapter One

What Is *Maharishi Ayur-Veda* Health Care?

When I first heard about Maharishi Ayur-Veda health care,[1] what appealed to me was that it made such good sense— such good, ordinary, everyday common sense. It was like the wise voice of my grandmother, telling me to how to take care of myself and stay healthy—or like the accumulated wisdom of all the grandmothers in the world collected into one supreme tradition of practical knowledge.

Once I had discovered this tradition, I could not get enough of it. It was like coming back home. Every new layer of knowledge felt comfortable, like discovering a layer of my own self.

Like others of my generation, I grew up in a traditional Indian household. But as I studied for a medical degree, went on to specialize in anesthesiology, left for the United States and started my practice as a physician, the comfortable feeling of "home" seemed very far away. It was easy to forget the simple routines that keep life healthy and happy. Discovering the Maharishi Ayur-Veda approach was a vivid reminder of all that was really valuable and important in my life.

Like the wisdom of grandmothers handed down through the generations, Maharishi Ayur-Veda health care was not invented yesterday. It is, in fact, the oldest tradition of health care in the world. However, its full glory was hidden from view for many generations.

It is due to the efforts and attention of Maharishi Mahesh Yogi that the entire knowledge is available in this day and age. Before

---

[1] Please note that, throughout the book, wherever "I" is used, it refers to Dr. Reddy's personal experience as a physician.

5

Maharishi, the knowledge had lost its firm footing in the practical knowledge of how to develop consciousness. Ayur-Veda became known as just another kind of herbal medicine. But Maharishi collected around him the greatest living exponents of the knowledge, delved deep into the classical texts of Ayur-Veda, and brought the tradition to life. Now the Maharishi Ayur-Veda system again offers complete health care, complete knowledge of life, as it was originally cognized by the great seers, or "Maharishis" of the ancient Vedic civilization.

Maharishi Mahesh Yogi is known worldwide as the founder of the Transcendental Meditation® program and its advanced programs, which he has been teaching around the world since 1957. He has also started Maharishi Universities of Management, Maharishi Vedic Universities and Maharishi Ayur-Veda Universities in the United States and around the world.

Maharishi Ayur-Veda health care is part of the complete Maharishi Vedic Approach to Health℠ program. *Veda* simply means "knowledge." The Maharishi Vedic Approach to Health is based on knowledge—complete knowledge about life and the laws of nature that govern living.

"Complete" means that nothing is left out. The Maharishi Ayur-Veda program takes care of every level of life—spiritual, mental, emotional, physical, behavioral. It creates health for the individual, health for society as a whole, health for the environment, and health for the entire universe. From the very smallest to the very largest—this is the range of Maharishi Ayur-Veda health care.

On a personal level, discovering this tradition was like coming back home. But on a professional level, as a physician, discovering the Maharishi Ayur-Veda approach was like opening the door to a whole new world. Its detailed, systematic and complete knowledge about prevention especially impressed me. The classical texts of Ayur-Veda cover all major branches of modern medicine, but the special attention given to preventive health care truly expanded my horizons. Modern medicine simply has nothing like it.

6

I realized immediately that here was something that filled a major gap in my medical education. And I knew immediately that, with this knowledge, I truly had something valuable to give my patients.

Many Approaches

The Maharishi Ayur-Veda program offers many different approaches for the prevention and treatment of disease.

First and foremost is the Transcendental Meditation technique. The practice of this simple, natural, effortless procedure carries with it profound benefits for health, as has been demonstrated by over 500 scientific studies. Some of these studies are included in chapter eighteen, and chapter eight provides more information about the technique itself.

Secondly, there are therapies that utilize the body to create health. For example, each of the five senses can be used as a powerful way to balance the overall functioning of the mind and body. Vedic exercises and specific patterns of breathing can also be therapeutic in different ways. A program of seasonal rejuvenation, which includes the application of herbalized oils, gentle heat treatments and elimination therapies, is another profound approach because it purifies the body of accumulated toxins.

Diet, when tailored to a person's individual needs, can create health, as can the specific application of plants and minerals. The literature of the Maharishi Ayur-Veda tradition includes a complete classification of herbs according to their therapeutic value. In addition, specialized herbal preparations called *rasayanas* maximize vitality, promote longevity, increase mental clarity and support the growth of consciousness.

One of the most beautiful aspects of the Maharishi Ayur-Veda approach, to my way of thinking, is the detailed knowledge of biological and environmental rhythms, which translates into specific daily and seasonal routines for maximizing health. These natural routines of life make the experience of living more effortless, as if nature were "on our side" working to accomplish our desires. When

7

we live in tune with natural law, there is less wear and tear, less resistance to our daily activity. The precious knowledge of how behavior can be used to balance life and create ideal health is unique to this system. More information about the Maharishi Ayur-Veda behavioral approach can be found in chapter eleven.

Pulse diagnosis is another beautiful aspect. With Maharishi Ayur-Veda pulse diagnosis, a physician can identify the nature of any imbalance which is responsible for existing symptoms of disease, as well as any subtle imbalance that might lead to disease over time. Pulse diagnosis is therapeutic in and of itself, and is central to the prevention strategies of the Maharishi Ayur-Veda approach. Maharishi Ayur-Veda Universities and Schools also provide courses for the public on self-pulse reading, so that everyone can learn to evaluate his or her own pulse and take appropriate measures to prevent or treat imbalances.

Maharishi Ayur-Veda knowledge addresses more than the individual. This tradition recognizes that society is a natural extension of the individual, and that influences in the environment have a powerful effect upon the health of the individual. Therefore, the Maharishi Ayur-Veda system also prescribes specific procedures and therapies to correct unhealthy trends in society and the world around us.

Primary among these approaches is the group practice of the Transcendental Meditation and TM-Sidhi® programs (the TM-Sidhi program, including Yogic Flying, is an advanced program of the Transcendental Meditation technique) which effectively dissolves stress and creates coherence in the collective consciousness of society as a whole. The Maharishi Ayur-Veda tradition also offers complete and detailed knowledge of how to build homes, plan cities and towns, and locate ourselves in our natural environment so that we take advantage of natural law. Environments that are noisy, polluted, congested, violent and full of fear are not conducive for living long, healthy lives. The knowledge of how to structure our environment for health is another precious aspect of this age-old system of natural health care.

Our extended environment is the universe around us—other planets, the sun, stars and distant galaxies. The Maharishi Ayur-Veda tradition offers the Vedic science of prediction—the Maharishi Jyotish℠ program—to deal with this distant environment. Through Maharishi Jyotish consultations we can identify the risk factors that make us vulnerable to certain diseases and take proper precautions to avert the danger that has not yet come.

There is much more about these approaches in the chapters that follow. But in this introductory chapter, we wanted to give you a brief overview, a glimpse of possibilities. This is just the beginning!

Highlights from History

Before we look ahead, let's look back—at the past few years of record achievement. Maharishi Ayur-Veda health care has come a long way in a very short time, since it was reintroduced to the world by Maharishi.

In 1985, Maharishi formulated his "World Plan for Perfect Health." This was a comprehensive strategy to bring success to the health care systems of every nation through Maharishi Ayur-Veda programs. It provided a master plan for the establishment of research centers, the training of physicians, technicians, pharmacists and agronomists, the cultivation of medicinal plants, the manufacture of natural herbal remedies, and the establishment of health centers and health education programs around the world.

You can see that, right from the beginning, Maharishi recognized the potential of the Maharishi Ayur-Veda approach—and he did not hesitate to apply it on a global scale!

In 1986, Maharishi initiated a global campaign to create a disease-free society through Maharishi Ayur-Veda programs. This campaign was begun during the months of October and November of 1986 and succeeded from the start in bringing this tradition to the attention of the media and leaders in the health care industry all over the world.

In the next few years, more than a thousand medical doctors were trained in the practice of Maharishi Ayur-Veda health care.

These doctors returned to their communities and started offering new Maharishi Ayur-Veda knowledge and therapies to their patients. The results were always gratifying.

At the same time, regional Maharishi Ayur-Veda Medical Centers were opened throughout the United States and the world. These centers offered in-house rejuvenation treatments, and made Maharishi Ayur-Veda health care available to anyone who could travel. Thousands of patients who had no local doctor trained in the Maharishi Ayur-Veda approach took advantage of the opportunity.

Maharishi Ayur-Veda Products International, Inc. was also established to provide traditional herbal formulas. Prepared exactly as described in the age-old texts, these formulas nourish and strengthen the entire mind-body system while they correct fundamental imbalances.

The idea in the beginning was to make "Maharishi Ayur-Veda" a household word. Maharishi felt that everyone should know about it and have the opportunity to create ideal health for themselves and their families. Ten years ago this seemed an almost impossible dream.

But it turned out to be visionary. Today Maharishi Ayur-Veda health care is well-known and well-respected around the world, and millions of people have benefited from it. The most powerful tool in making the dream a reality turned out to be word of mouth. If something makes a practical difference in peoples' lives—it gets around!

Health education programs were part of Maharishi's plan right from the beginning. Now a full range of courses is available for everyone at local branches of Maharishi Ayur-Veda Universities and Schools. As of the writing of this book, there is also a strong move to establish Maharishi Colleges of Vedic Medicine around the world that will offer undergraduate and graduate degree programs in this new approach.

Research on Maharishi Ayur-Veda therapies has been ongoing. Since 1970, hundreds of studies have demonstrated the beneficial effects of the Transcendental Meditation technique alone, and in the past ten years, studies have also examined other Maharishi Ayur-Veda approaches. These studies, taken as a whole, show remarkable improvement in the health of the participants—as measured objectively and experienced subjectively. Hari Sharma, M.D. of The Ohio State University conducted many of the breakthrough studies showing the effects of Maharishi Ayur-Veda herbal formulas on free radicals. This research, and its implications for health care, were published in his book *Freedom from Disease* (Veda Publishing, Toronto, Canada, 1993). Commenting on the Maharishi Ayur-Veda approach, Dr. Sharma said, "I believe we are in the midst of a medical revolution, the type that occurs only once every hundred years or so." We discuss the topic of free radicals and Dr. Sharma's research more thoroughly in chapter seven.

One of the most exciting developments in research has been the work of physician and neuroscientist Tony Nader, M.D., Ph.D., who is International President of Maharishi Ayur-Veda Universities. Dr. Nader looked closely at the physical structure of the human physiology in the light of Maharishi's teachings and insights into ancient Vedic Literature. He discovered an exact correlation (in both structure and function) between specific areas of the human physiology and the various aspects of the Veda and Vedic Literature. This discovery suggests that the human body is an exact replica of the fundamental laws of nature expressed in the Veda and Vedic Literature—which are the same laws of nature that govern the universe. Dr. Nader feels that the discovery of this correlation "raises the individual dignity of human beings to the cosmic dignity of the universe." He has described his findings in his book *Human Physiology: Expression of Veda and the Vedic Literature* (Maharishi Vedic University Press, Vlodrop, The Netherlands, 1994).

As a physician, it is reassuring to have the support of a worldwide Maharishi Ayur-Veda organization and a network of colleagues, many of them engaged in research. With the support of Maharishi Ayur-Veda Medical Centers, Maharishi Ayur-Veda Universities, Maharishi Ayur-Veda™ products, and my medical colleagues around the world, I feel completely confident applying Maharishi Ayur-Veda therapies in my private practice. And I know that wherever my patients go, they can receive the education and support that they need to create ideal health using the Maharishi Ayur-Veda approach.

On one level, Maharishi Ayur-Veda health care is all about everyday common sense. But on another level, its traditional knowledge expands our boundaries and changes the way we think. "Perfect health," "disease-free society," "cosmic dignity of the universe"—these are not phrases usually associated with health care. But the health care most of us have received for most of our lives is actually "disease care." The knowledge of how to create and maintain health has been missing. Now that knowledge is at hand. And it turns out to be the oldest knowledge of all, timeless and time-proven—now fully restored for the needs of a modern age.

Summary

The Maharishi Ayur-Veda system is the world's oldest and most comprehensive system of natural health care. Now restored to its full value by Maharishi Mahesh Yogi, it offers complete knowledge of life and how to create and maintain an ideal state of health.

Chapter Two

Health: Old and New Perspectives

The word "health" comes from the Indo-European root *kailo* meaning "whole." As defined by the World Health Organization, health is "a state of complete physical, mental and social well-being and not merely the absence of disease or infirmity." According to the classical texts of Ayur-Veda, a healthy person will be one whose physiology is integrated and balanced, and whose self, mind and senses remain full of bliss.

But how many people actually experience this kind of health? Unfortunately, most people have a completely different view. Let this diagram illustrate the range of health, on a scale of 0 to 100:

0	50	100

Extreme illness or death is represented by 0 and total health or well-being by 100. The midpoint of 50 represents a blend of illness and wellness. At this midpoint we are neither totally ill nor totally well.

As we go through life, most people experience their health as fluctuating between periods of moderate or even severe illness (25) and periods of relative comfort and ease (75), on either side of the midpoint (50):

0	25	50	75	100

Discomforts such as headaches and PMS, debilitating aches and pains, allergies, and illnesses such as colds, flu and occasional viruses are accepted as a normal part of the human experience within this range.

Below the midpoint we experience severe illness and disease. We turn to drugs, surgery or other therapies in an attempt to feel relatively healthier. It's common to feel helplessly at the mercy of our disease.

0	25	50	75	100

Above the midpoint and free of debilitating symptoms, we experience a condition of relative comfort and ease, consider ourselves blessed or lucky, and say that we are "healthy."

0	25	50	75	100

I think most of us can relate to this model of health. And we accept it as the norm because we feel we don't have a choice. We want good health, but to a large extent feel it's out of our personal control.

This book was written to let you know that there is a choice, that there is a better way. According to the Maharishi Ayur-Veda tradition, human life span can be extended well beyond what is commonly accepted as normal, and you should expect to live every day of your life in vibrant, radiant health. Using the knowledge and natural approaches of Maharishi Ayur-Veda health care, it's possible to take command of your life and create perfect health. The experience of a growing number of people using the Maharishi Ayur-Veda approach in their daily lives verifies this. It's possible to enjoy, not only freedom from disease, but a positive and permanent state of well-being.

Maharishi Ayur-Veda health care makes possible the impossible by eliminating the underlying causes of disease. As the root problem is corrected, it's natural to feel healthier and happier. Illnesses strike less often; immune system functioning grows stronger; periods of health last longer. The growth is cumulative and it accelerates over time.

Using the practical knowledge of Maharishi Ayur-Veda health care, it's possible to move from a compromised, ever-changing state of health to an absolute and invincible state of health and happiness. In the following chapters we will explain how.

Summary

Most people understand health to mean "relatively free from disease." With Maharishi Ayur-Veda health care, we can experience health as wholeness—complete and blissful well-being.

Chapter Three

Beyond Symptoms

How many times have you reached for a tablet to ease the pain of a headache, heartburn, or insomnia? When you're suffering, it's natural to want relief.

However, if you jump to the conclusion that symptoms are the cause of your disease, and that symptomatic relief is as good as a cure, you are definitely "putting the cart before the horse." Instant relief should not be confused with solving the underlying problem. When you choose Maharishi Ayur-Veda health care, you choose to get to the source of your problem. In this chapter we will describe how, with the Maharishi Ayur-Veda approach, you can eliminate the root cause of your disease.

Symptoms Are Not the Cause

Conventional medicine specializes in treating symptoms. If you have a cold, you take antihistamines. If you have an infection, you take antibiotics. If you have a growth here or there, you cut it out. An amazing range of "cures" is available for almost every symptom of disease. But there is not enough knowledge about how and why the symptom occurred in the first place, and how to prevent its recurrence.

That is why many of us experience one set of symptoms after another. The underlying weakness remains in the body and gives rise to the same or new symptoms over and over, trapping us in an endless cycle of sickness and temporary recovery. For example, a common cold leads to bronchitis, which leads to a sinus infection, which then affects the ears. And just when you think you're finally better, you catch another cold!

A more serious example is cancer. How many patients have a malignant growth removed surgically, only to develop another?

The great strength of the Maharishi Ayur-Veda system is that it can identify and correct the fundamental imbalance that causes the disease in the first place. With Maharishi Ayur-Veda health care, symptoms disappear, not because they are suppressed or removed, but because the body is returned to its own natural state of health.

Working with the Body's Inner Intelligence

Conventional medicine views the body as a complicated collection of parts (heart, kidneys, brain, lymphatic system, digestive system, etc.) and treats it as if it were a mechanical wind-up toy only needing a new spring here, or a wheel adjusted there, to work properly. In contrast, Maharishi Ayur-Veda health care treats the entire person— mind, body, behavior and environment—as one continuous and interrelated whole, a whole that is more than the sum of its parts.

The Maharishi Ayur-Veda tradition wisely recognizes that within each of us is an innate intelligence that orchestrates and coordinates the virtually infinite number of "moving parts" that make up our body. This is the same natural intelligence that orchestrates and coordinates the entire universe. It is the same intelligent order that keeps the planets moving in their orbits, makes the seasons come on time, and prevents an apple or a peach from growing on a pear tree.

Maharishi Ayur-Veda therapies strengthen the entire physiology from within by gently enlivening this natural intelligence. When intelligence is lively we are in balance, and symptoms disappear. As our physiology gains strength and flexibility, we develop a natural resistance to disease.

Maharishi Ayur-Veda health care works to eliminate the cause of disease—underlying imbalances. With the application of Maharishi Ayur-Veda therapies, some symptoms may be relieved faster than others, depending on the severity and duration of the underlying imbalance, but the emphasis is always on correcting the fundamental cause of disease. In this way, when the symptoms disappear, they disappear for good.

Your Personalized Guidelines

Your physician will work with you to develop your personal Maharishi Ayur-Veda program for better health. This program will include suggestions for diet, your daily routine, what kind of exercise (if any) would be helpful, the use of herbal supplements, and techniques for the elimination of stress. It may also include recommendations for other therapies, depending on your unique situation. Your program is always individualized according to your personal needs and lifestyle, and also according to the environment and season of the year.

From your side, all that is needed is the sincere desire to get well. In fact, the patient's intention to get better is one of the most important and powerful ingredients in the healing process. It's your contribution, and, if strong, it alone can effect a cure—as suggested by numerous documented cases of unexplained, spontaneous cures.

It's also important to take the time to allow your new program to work. Following your Maharishi Ayur-Veda recommendations is like having a road map. The map shows the way to your destination and guides you there, step by step, turn by turn. It may take time, but progress is assured.

Your destination is total health, and it is not only attainable, it is your birthright! It's never too late to claim a birthright. Using the Maharishi Ayur-Veda health care system as your guide, you can effortlessly claim what was yours all along.

Summary

Maharishi Ayur-Veda health care addresses not just the symptom, but the underlying imbalance that caused the symptom. Working with the body's own natural intelligence, it corrects the imbalance and returns the physiology to a natural state of vibrant health.

19

Chapter Four

Safe, Simple, Effective

Historically, there is no medical science on earth that has withstood the test of time for as long as Ayur-Veda. It predates written history, and basic principles of Ayur-Veda can be found in ancient Greek medicine as well as other ancient systems of medicine. Ayur-Veda served the needs of hundreds of millions of people from the time of the Vedic civilization until the occupation of the Indian subcontinent during the late Middle Ages. At that time, other systems of medicine gained prominence and Ayur-Veda was lost from view.

Thanks to the efforts and insight of Maharishi Mahesh Yogi, the entire body of knowledge is again available. The Maharishi Ayur-Veda system of health care is the knowledge of Ayur-Veda restored to its original purity. Development of consciousness is again understood to be of primary importance in creating ideal health. All Maharishi Ayur-Veda approaches work because they enliven our own inner intelligence—pure consciousness.

We've all noticed that health fads and crazes have their day in the sun, but are soon replaced by new fads and crazes. What has limited value lasts for a limited time. Maharishi Ayur-Veda therapies have passed the test of time because they work on a deeper level. They are safe, simple—and very effective.

Safe

Maharishi Ayur-Veda therapies are safe because they work holistically. They treat the whole person, not just a part. For example, an herbal formula given to help the skin might also strengthen digestion and nourish the immune system at the same time. This is because the herbs address a fundamental imbalance that affects all three areas. Because of this holistic advantage, it's common for patients to happily report unexpected "side benefits" from taking Maharishi Ayur-Veda herbal formulas.

Moreover, the tradition uses combinations of whole herbs, not isolated, so-called "active ingredients" that often result in harmful side effects.

This is just one example of how Maharishi Ayur-Veda health care provides for patient safety. Side effects and safety are important issues, especially today when it is estimated that 25% of all disease is a direct side effect of modern-day conventional treatment. Hospitals are the best place to catch an infectious disease, and hospital-bred strains are hard to control because of their immunity to standard treatment. Instead of the disease-free society envisioned a couple of generations ago with the discovery of antibiotics, we are now facing the spectre of new and even more deadly strains of disease.

A precept of Ayur-Veda is that medicine should cure without causing any additional disease or negative side effect. Maharishi Ayur-Veda health care delivers just this kind of ideal treatment.

Simple

Maharishi Ayur-Veda therapies are simple because they are natural. They work with nature and the body's own inner intelligence to accomplish the goal. For example, your physician might recommend that you eat your biggest meal at midday because it is easier for your system to digest at that time. Or your doctor may suggest that you wake up with the sun, so you can take advantage of the liveliness available only in the early morning hours. These simple lifestyle changes actually fine-tune your natural biological rhythms to work more efficiently with nature and create better health from the inside out.

Likewise, using diet to create better health is very important in the Maharishi Ayur-Veda system. This is because the food we eat supplies not only necessary calories and nutrition, but also the lively value of nature's intelligence that nourishes our bodies on a deeper level. We've all heard the saying, "You are what you eat." Eating proper food is a powerful way to help correct imbalances and promote health. And what could be simpler or more natural than eating good food?

Of course, your physician will make personalized recommendations for your diet, daily routine and other therapies based on your individual needs. For example, one person would benefit from hot, spicy food; another should avoid hot spices altogether. One patient should make vigorous daily exercise a priority; for another, a leisurely walk two or three times a week is ideal.

Effective

Maharishi Ayur-Veda therapies are effective because they work on deeper, more powerful levels of the mind and body. In the previous chapter we described how this system of health care deals not just with symptoms, but with the underlying causes of disease. It works with the body's intelligence to correct imbalances, strengthen the physiology and prevent future disorders.

On the deepest level of the mind and body is pure consciousness, or pure intelligence. All Maharishi Ayur-Veda therapies enliven this most fundamental level. It's like watering the root of a tree—the whole tree flourishes.

The simple effortless procedure of the Transcendental Meditation (TM®) technique gives the direct experience of pure consciousness, and because of this, is considered to be the first and foremost approach of the Maharishi Ayur-Veda program. The daily practice of the TM technique is the most effective way to develop your body's inner intelligence, and the most direct and effective way to improve your health as a whole. (There is more about the benefits of this technique in chapter eight.)

In addition, your physician will often recommend the TM technique because it is extremely effective in eliminating stress, one of the major factors contributing to disease.

For Your Peace of Mind

Health professionals know that medical treatments have different kinds of value. They have *perceived* value (what everyone in the situation thinks and feels about the treatment), *quantifiable* value (what can be measured about the treatment in scientific tests), and *subjective* value (what the patient being treated actually experiences). All of these values are important, but they are not equally important.

A therapy or drug can be studied, analyzed, and tested scientifically, but the ultimate validation is always the experience of the user over time. With conventional modern medicine, new drugs and new procedures are tested for only a limited length of time before they are considered "safe" for distribution. Although they have not been widely available, some Ayur-Veda therapies— including the use of herbal formulas—have been in continuous use for thousands of years.

There is no more important test than the test of time. Even after a modern drug has passed all the tests required by the pharmaceutical industry and government regulatory agencies, there is still a risk—and that risk is unknown. Just recall the tragic circumstances surrounding the release of the drug thalidomide a generation ago. Supposedly a "safe" treatment for morning sickness, it resulted in a high percentage of birth defects and daughters who developed uterine cancer. This is just one example of a drug, untested by time, that caused untold suffering.

With Maharishi Ayur-Veda health care you are building on the experience of countless generations before you. There is nothing "new" in the Maharishi Ayur-Veda approach—just time-tested, time-proven therapies that have real value in preventing disease and restoring health. There are no risks, no hidden side effects, no surprises—only the best that history has to offer.

One more point for your peace of mind: only licensed physicians administer Maharishi Ayur-Veda health care. In addition to their modern medical training, these doctors receive specialized training in prevention and the diagnosis and treatment of disease using the Maharishi Ayur-Veda approach. These physicians understand and appreciate contemporary medicine, but they want to give their patients the safest, easiest and most effective care possible. This inspired their decision to go on for more, the "more" that is available only with the Maharishi Ayur-Veda approach. With the attention of these physicians, patients benefit from the best of both worlds, and receive the finest, most complete, most natural health care on earth.

Summary

Maharishi Ayur-Veda health care is ideal for everyone. It is safe, simple, natural, effective, time-proven and complete.

Chapter Five

Benefits for Everyone

Ayur-Vedo Amritanam—Ayur-Veda is for those who desire
immortality.   *—Charaka Samhita*

After twenty years in crisis-oriented medicine, it's heartwarming
for me to be working now as a family physician. My favorite
patients are the ones who are not yet born! With their mothers
following the safe, gentle techniques of the Maharishi Ayur-Veda
program, I feel these lucky children are entering the world with a
huge head start.

The primary focus of Maharishi Ayur-Veda health care is the
prevention of disease, and it's never too early to start. From the
moment of conception, through birth, infancy, childhood,
adolescence, adulthood and old age, the Maharishi Ayur-Veda
tradition provides knowledge and guidelines for how to create and
maintain balance so that symptoms of disease need never arise. The
guidelines are always easy to follow, because they are natural. They
simply remind us how to live naturally, in tune with ourselves and
our environment.

Prevention, Treatment, Promotion of Health

If you are blessed with good health, Maharishi Ayur-Veda health
care will help you maintain it—and teach you how to make it stronger
and more invincible. If you suffer from one ailment or another, then
Maharishi Ayur-Veda therapies will treat the underlying imbalance
that caused the problem. All conditions can be helped, because
Maharishi Ayur-Veda treatments attack the very root of the disease.

As a physician, I have many patients who have come to me with
so-called "chronic" disorders—such as chronic fatigue, persistent
allergies, irritable bowel syndrome, arthritis, lower back pain,

27

sinusitis, skin disorders, hypertension, weight gain or loss, sleep disorders, substance abuse, anxiety or depression, menstrual or menopause problems, or migraine headaches. In my experience, I have found that these chronic disorders respond well to the Maharishi Ayur-Veda approach, or a combination of Maharishi Ayur-Veda treatment and conventional care.

As people grow older, one out of three can now expect to be affected by a chronic degenerative disease. With Maharishi Ayur-Veda health care we finally have a system that can help prevent the occurrence of these diseases, and provide relief for those who have them.

Even patients who have multiple sclerosis, other neuromuscular disorders, cancer, AIDS, or combined ailments will benefit by a correction of underlying imbalances and improved immunity to disease. For these patients, Maharishi Ayur-Veda therapies are used in conjunction with conventional medicine.

Rejuvenation

The benefits to health that come with using the Maharishi Ayur-Veda approach have been examined by the scientific community and the results published in dozens of professional journals. These scientific studies document improved general health—improved digestion, sleep, energy, state of mind, resistance to illness—as well as improvement in specific diseases such as asthma and heart disease. (See chapter eighteen.)

Furthermore, studies document an overall trend toward biological youthfulness. Using certain parameters (such as near-point vision, auditory threshold and blood pressure) to determine "biological age," studies have found that patients who use Maharishi Ayur-Veda health care have a significantly younger biological age than control groups and the general population. (See page 159.)

I often tease my patients and tell them they are getting younger by the minute—and with Maharishi Ayur-Veda health care, that is the truth! Increased vitality, youthfulness, and feelings of freedom, spontaneity and joy are commonly experienced by my patients. As their doctor, I can see it written on their faces, and feel it in their pulse.

The studies verify what we can expect from Maharishi Ayur-Veda health care—prevention of disease, promotion of better health, treatment for serious and chronic complaints, a better quality of life and improved longevity. Using this system of natural health care we can look forward to the joy of living in a healthy body even in our most advanced years. Our "golden years" can truly be golden.

Summary

No matter what your age or state of health, the Maharishi Ayur-Veda system has something to offer. From birth to old age, from serious disease to total wellness, Maharishi Ayur-Veda health care provides knowledge and experience to bring fullness to life.

Chapter Six

How *Maharishi Ayur-Veda* Health Care Complements Conventional Medicine

Ayur-Veda is that simple, natural program for perfect health that eliminates all imbalances—in the physiology, psychology, behavior, and environment. All the different health systems of the world are going to be fulfilled with support and enrichment from Ayur-Veda.   —Maharishi Mahesh Yogi

It wasn't too long ago that, for health care, there was just one family doctor who, with unquestioned authority, handled all the family health needs from birth to death. From my own childhood I have vivid memories of "the doctor," stethoscope around his neck and black bag in hand, who took care of everything. He even made house calls to feverish children, and often stayed on to chat for a few minutes with the family.

This familiar, almost stereotypical figure is fading fast from most cultures, as is the reliance on one doctor for all the family's needs. Today is the era of specialists, and it is more common for a family to have half a dozen doctors that they see regularly.

The reliance on one system of medicine is also a thing of the past. As East traveled West, and the globe became an oversized village, an increasing range of health care options became available, no matter where one happened to live. Patients who were dissatisfied with their care sought better service elsewhere, or felt free to mix and match as they pleased. And with the dawn of the "new age" came an explosion of alternative therapies.

The system of medicine accepted by most developed countries today as "conventional" includes: immunization, prescription drug therapy, vitamin and mineral supplements, surgical procedures, chemical and radiation therapies, and in extreme cases, the life-support systems available in hospitals. Chiropractic and osteopathic spinal manipulation are also increasingly accepted as conventional. For diseases considered "mental," modern medicine offers counseling, psychoanalysis and behavior modification, as well as the use of chemicals.

Experience has shown that most systems of medicine, both conventional and unconventional, have some value. Certain methods of treatment seem to work better in some cultures than in others. A few methods seem to work in all cultures, but are not practical for worldwide application because of cost or other factors.

When we think about health care we tend to think of the system that we ourselves know and accept, from our own cultural backgrounds and personal experience. Unfortunately, we also tend to dismiss health technologies that we don't know or haven't experienced.

The limitations of our current systems of health care are obvious, since no country can demonstrate total health, either for its citizens or for society as a whole. Even conventional health care, while very successful in some ways, is unable to address many fundamental concerns—such as the need for effective prevention of disease and for treatment of the root causes of disease.

The Maharishi Ayur-Veda tradition offers what has been missing: a complete system of natural medicine that aims to create total health. Its therapies are simple, natural, and effective for everyone. And because it emphasizes prevention rather than cure, Maharishi Ayur-Veda health care is extremely cost-effective, making it practical for worldwide use.

It may not be the system of medicine we remember from our childhood—but it's "just what the doctor ordered." And with its emphasis on well-care we may soon be back to the comforting image of a family physician making regular house calls—just to check in on healthy, happy patients.

From My Own Experience

I speak from experience when I say that the Maharishi Ayur-Veda approach can work hand in hand very successfully with other systems of medicine. It need not replace what we already have; it can beautifully complement what a patient is already using. It's the "something more" that we all want and need.

I have often worked closely with a patient's primary care doctor—another licensed M.D. or health care specialist—to provide for my patient's best interest. I have recommended conventional therapies such as prescription drugs or surgery, when I feel that is necessary. Often there is a transition time, when patients continue with their old regimen, but add Maharishi Ayur-Veda therapies at the same time. As the physiology grows stronger, I often decrease the dose, or eliminate the use of prescription medicines altogether. In addition, patients experience fewer side effects from conventional treatment when they incorporate Maharishi Ayur-Veda therapies; for example, patients undergoing chemotherapy or radiation report less of the discomfort usually associated with radical treatments.

When a patient chooses to use Maharishi Ayur-Veda health care in conjunction with conventional medicine or other therapies, everyone benefits. The patients receive the best care available, the "best of both worlds," while strengthening their systems to prevent future disease. The patients' primary care physicians learn how to broaden their healing approach and gain the satisfaction that comes from helping their patients get better. The physicians practicing the Maharishi Ayur-Veda approach enjoy the fulfillment that comes from seeing patients grow toward total health, with the added satisfaction of sharing with their colleagues information about this age-old system of health care.

The best part is the joy and happiness of the patients, who have lived with the disease and now feel more in control of their health.

Patients who have not responded to conventional treatment, or who have suffered from chronic ailments for years without finding relief, or who are tired of depending on medication year in and year out are especially delighted with the results. Other patients, who have experienced irritating, uncomfortable, or even debilitating side effects from conventional medicine, appreciate the safety of the Maharishi Ayur-Veda approach. And patients with so-called incurable or terminal diseases are grateful for the opportunity to dramatically improve their quality of living, as well as their state of health. With Maharishi Ayur-Veda health care, we all have the opportunity to add not only "years to our lives," but also "life to our years."

Summary

Maharishi Ayur-Veda health care supplies what has been missing in conventional medicine and other healing technologies. With the addition of this approach, all doctors can offer complete health care to their patients.

How *Maharishi Ayur-Veda* Health Care Complements Conventional Medicine	
What Conventional Medicine Offers:	**What *Maharishi Ayur-Veda* Health Care Adds:**
Prevention	
• Immunization for childhood diseases, tuberculosis, influenza and other infectious illnesses	• Complete knowledge and practical guidelines for maintaining balance for life-long health
• Balanced diet according to major food groups and recommended daily allowances; regular exercise	• Specific guidelines for diet and exercise based on each person's individual needs
• Vitamin and mineral supplements	• Holistic herbal formulas (such as Maharishi Amrit Kalash™ Nectar and Ambrosia) to improve immunity to disease and develop higher states of consciousness
• Lifestyle changes such as no smoking, less alcohol	• Techniques (such as the practice of the Transcendental Meditation technique) that help negative habits drop away naturally and permanently, without effort

What Conventional Medicine Offers:	What *Maharishi Ayur-Veda* Health Care Adds:
Diagnosis of Disease	
• Evaluation of symptoms	• Pulse diagnosis to determine underlying imbalances that cause symptoms of existing or forthcoming disease (see chapter fourteen)
• Tests to determine the nature of the disease	• Less dependence on expensive, invasive testing procedures; more reliance on getting to know each patient and his or her needs
• Documentation of personal and family history to help identify risk factors	• Identification of future risk factors for forthcoming imbalances or diseases through the Vedic science of prediction (the Maharishi Jyotish program; see chapter nineteen)

What Conventional Medicine Offers:	What *Maharishi Ayur-Veda* Health Care Adds:
Treatment	
• Prescription drugs and over-the-counter drugs for the alleviation of symptoms of disease	• Diagnosis and treatment of the underlying imbalance that caused the disease so that symptoms disappear on their own; nourishing therapies that reduce side effects from taking drugs
• Antibiotics for fighting bacterial infections	• Therapies and herbs that strengthen the immune system to resist infection naturally
• Radical treatments such as surgery, chemotherapy and radiation	• Nourishing herbs and other therapies that complement by minimizing the discomfort and side effects associated with radical treatments, and help the body recover from them
• Setting of broken bones, stitches for open wounds, other surgical procedures	• Herbs and other therapies that complement by helping broken bones and wounds heal more completely and efficiently

What Conventional Medicine Offers:	What *Maharishi Ayur-Veda* Health Care Adds:
Treatment (continued)	
• Acute care and life-saving intervention for serious accidents and emergencies	• Techniques (such as the practice of the TM technique) that eliminate stress and help prevent serious disease; other therapies that relieve the trauma of stressful situations
• Hospital life-support systems	• Techniques and therapies to improve the quality of life
• For mental disorders: counseling, psycho-analysis, behavior modification, and drug therapy	• Holistic therapies that treat the mind, body, behavior and environment as one interrelated whole; techniques to balance the emotions and develop higher states of consciousness; herbs to nourish and balance the entire mind-body system
Rejuvenation	
• Vacations for a change of pace	• Guidelines for living a balanced routine of life day in and day out (cont.)

What Conventional Medicine Offers:	What *Maharishi Ayur-Veda* Health Care Adds:
Rejuvenation (continued)	
	(including the practice of the TM technique for a twice-daily "mini-vacation"); seasonal rejuvenation therapies to eliminate toxins and refresh the entire mind-body system; techniques and therapies that reverse the aging process and improve the quality of life
Global Health	
• Public education programs to curb the spread of disease and raise public awareness about how to protect our natural environment	• Complete and detailed knowledge about how to prevent disease and create life-long health, including the Maharishi Sthapatya Veda[SM] program, the Vedic science of architecture and environmental planning, to ensure that our environment does not create the ground for imbalance and disease (see chapter nineteen)

What Conventional Medicine Offers:	What *Maharishi Ayur-Veda* Health Care Adds:
Global Health (continued)	
• Governmental regulation of food and drugs to ensure safety for the consumer; international agreements to improve the quality of our environment	• Techniques and programs (such as the group practice of the TM and TM-Sidhi programs) that purify the environment, reduce social stress, cut violent crime, improve governmental effective-ness, raise collective consciousness, and create a better quality of life for all

Chapter Seven

The Root Causes of Disease

This chapter answers the big question in every patient's mind—
"Why?" Why me? Why this disease? Why this pain and this
suffering at this time?

According to the Maharishi Ayur-Veda system of health care,
there are no mysterious causes of disease. This timeless tradition
provides not only complete knowledge about disease—why this
particular disorder in this particular patient at this particular time—
but also practical therapies to treat the root cause of disease and
restore each patient to health.

On the grossest, most obvious level of functioning, the root cause
of disease is the accumulation of impurities, or toxins, in the body.
The traditional word for this is *ama*. Ama is largely the result of
improper diet and incomplete digestion, and it collects in the body
as a thick, sticky, indigestible waste matter. Ama isn't created
overnight, but as it accumulates over time it collects in your cells,
clogs your tissues, obstructs bodily channels and causes major
disruption on all levels of normal body functioning.

The personalized dietary guidelines that you receive from your
physician will help prevent the accumulation of ama and start to
cleanse the body of existing deposits. However, some general
guidelines that apply to everyone include avoiding food that has
unnatural additives and preservatives, and food that is aged,
fermented, left-over, highly processed or full of indigestible
ingredients. A variety of simple, fresh, wholesome, home-cooked
food is always best.

Another thing to keep in mind is that your digestive system works
most efficiently when it is given one meal at a time. Let your system
do the one job it has begun, before giving it more to do. The habit of
continuous eating or frequent snacking between meals will certainly

overload even the healthiest system and result in deposits of ama. Incomplete digestion of food, incomplete metabolism of nutrients, and incomplete elimination of waste products are all major causes of disease.

Arthritis is one disease that is directly linked to accumulation of ama in the joints. Cardiovascular disease results from ama blockage in arteries and veins. Menstrual disorders—such as PMS, fibroid tumors, infertility and endometriosis—are often related to deposits of ama in a woman's pelvic area. These are just a few examples of how ama can disrupt the body, causing gross symptoms of disease.

There is another kind of ama, which might be called "mental ama." Mental ama accumulates as a result of psychological stress, day-to-day problems, and experiencing negative emotions, such as anger, frustration, anxiety, depression and fear. These powerful emotions and the strains of everyday living have a direct effect on the body, and over time can cause major disturbances.

Fortunately, the Maharishi Ayur-Veda system of health care provides a complete range of therapies that effectively deal with all kinds of ama. Many of the approaches are preventive, such as eating a proper diet and following a good daily routine. Other approaches are preventive and therapeutic at the same time, such as the Maharishi Ayur-Veda seasonal rejuvenation program. Another example is the daily practice of the Transcendental Meditation technique, which rids the body of accumulated stress (both mental and physical) while it strengthens the entire mind-body system to work more efficiently.

Have You Heard about Free Radicals?

Ama is the traditional term for impurities that collect in the system and eventually disrupt its functioning. There is no equivalent concept in modern medical terminology. But the closest thing to it might be what scientists today are calling "free radicals." Free radicals are atoms or molecules that have at least one unpaired electron, making them highly volatile and reactive—and in the body, very damaging.

Free radicals are found everywhere, not just in our bodies. You see them at work in a car that's rusting, or in an apple that begins to turn brown and spoil once it has been cut. As a normal by-product of the oxidation process, free radicals are omnipresent in our oxygen-filled environment.

Oxidation and the formation of free radicals also occur naturally in bodily metabolism. These free radicals are no problem as long as the body can disarm them with its usual defenses. The problem comes when their numbers far exceed the body's ability to neutralize them. This is increasingly the case due to unhealthy environmental factors in today's world. Some scientists estimate that every cell in the body is now bombarded by 10,000 free radicals a day! There is no way that ordinary defenses can keep up with that kind of attack.

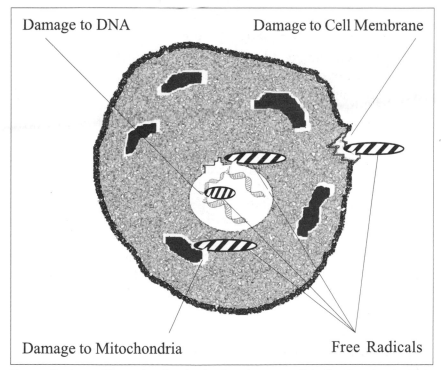

Damage to DNA Damage to Cell Membrane

Damage to Mitochondria Free Radicals

Free radicals are like molecular sharks that damage cell walls, the mitochondria (the cell's power plants) and the DNA (the cell's intelligence). All Maharishi Ayur-Veda therapies strengthen the body to resist the onslaught of free radicals.

Moreover, scientists estimate that astronomical numbers of free radicals are a contributing factor in over 70% of all disease—including atherosclerosis, rheumatoid arthritis, cancer, inflammatory bowel disease, Alzheimer's disease, depression of the immune system, and the degeneration associated with aging.[1]

If you never heard about free radicals in high school chemistry, I'm not surprised. Scientific attention on free radicals is a recent phenomenon; it has developed along with the factors that have contributed to their explosive growth. Scientists have isolated reasons for the explosion—and topping the list is the stress and strain of modern everyday living. Environmental pollution (toxins and pesticides in our air, water and food), poor diet, smoking, alcohol consumption, x-rays, radiation treatment and excessive exposure to the sun also increase free radical production.

Free radicals are, to a large extent, an inevitable by-product of living in the modern world. There's no avoiding them—but you can keep up with them and neutralize their harmful effects. All Maharishi Ayur-Veda therapies are effective in strengthening the body to resist the onslaught of free radicals. But one herbal combination in particular seems to have a remarkable and beneficial effect.

The name of this food supplement, containing 40 traditional herbs and fruits, is Maharishi Amrit Kalash. According to the Maharishi Ayur-Veda tradition, it nourishes the mind and body, increases immunity to disease, and supports the development of higher states of consciousness. As published research now documents, it also has an amazing power to fight free radicals. Studies show that it scavenges free radicals 1,000 times more effectively than other antioxidants (such as vitamin C, vitamin E and beta-carotene).

---

[1] For a thorough discussion of free radicals and the related research on Maharishi Ayur-Veda health care, I recommend a book by Hari Sharma, M.D. entitled *Freedom from Disease: How to Control Free Radicals, a Major Cause of Aging and Disease* (Veda Publishing, Inc., Suite 116, 65 Front Street West, Toronto, Ontario, Canada M5J 1E6).

Moreover, it is the only "full-spectrum" antioxidant, working both inside and outside the cell to eliminate the various kinds of free radicals.

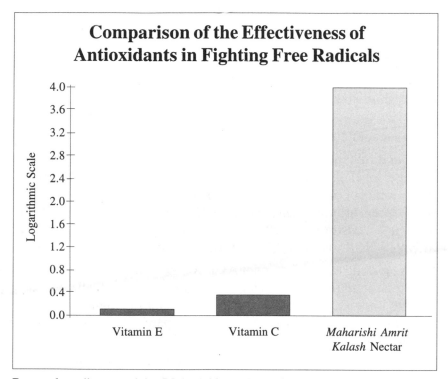

Comparison of the Effectiveness of Antioxidants in Fighting Free Radicals

Researchers discovered that Maharishi Amrit Kalash Nectar is 1,000 times more potent than vitamin C or E in neutralizing free radicals. The difference between them is so great that it can only be shown on the same chart by using a logarithmic scale on the vertical axis. (Reference: *Pharmacology, Biochemistry and Behavior* (43) 1992: 1175-1182.)

Research also indicates that the Maharishi Ayur-Veda seasonal rejuvenation program can eliminate free radicals from the body. In one study it was found that seasonal rejuvenation reduced serum lipid peroxide levels; that is, it reduced the number of fat molecules that had been damaged by free radicals. These fat molecules are thought to start the build-up of deposits in the arteries that leads to atherosclerosis and heart disease. The study also showed that vasoactive intestinal peptide (VIP) rose 80% after rejuvenation treatment—a very positive sign because VIP is responsible for dilating blood vessels and increasing blood flow to the heart.[2]

There is no mention of free radicals in the classical texts of Ayur-Veda. Yet the age-old formulas and therapies that are described there in detail continue to meet the challenges and health needs of each new generation. The traditional knowledge still applies—and is more timely than ever.

On a Deeper Level

Ama and free radicals contribute to disease on a gross level. But on a deeper level, there's more to it. Why, for example, does ama collect in the joints of one person, causing arthritis, while in another it gets deposited in arteries, causing atherosclerosis and heart disease? And why, in a classroom full of children catching the latest flu, is there always a handful of children who don't catch it at all?

According to the Maharishi Ayur-Veda tradition, there is always a reason for getting sick. And to understand the reason all you really need to understand is YOU!—and what inner imbalance made you vulnerable to a particular disorder at a particular time. There is nothing random about it at all.

Fortunately, the Maharishi Ayur-Veda system of health care provides all the knowledge you need to understand what caused the problem and how to solve it. The knowledge is detailed and accurate, and it's specific to each individual because no two people are alike. Your physician will be able to give you complete information about your situation, a program to correct imbalances, and guidelines to follow year-round to help maintain balance and ensure maximum health.

Once you know yourself and how to keep healthy, you'll know what works for you and what doesn't. For example, we all know

---

[2] *The Journal of Research and Education in Indian Medicine* 12 (1993): 3–13.

that "burning the midnight oil" night after night is bound to cause fatigue, and that it's easy to catch a cold if we don't dress warmly. These are common sense guidelines that apply to everyone. But the Maharishi Ayur-Veda system also provides individualized guidelines for diet, daily routine, type of exercise, choice of work and living environment. There is nothing about ourselves, our relationships with other people or our interaction with the environment that is not addressed.

The knowledge is complete—and it is also very simple. Underlying and supporting all the individual recommendations is the profound understanding that we're a part of nature, and we must live according to the natural laws that support health and well-being or face the consequences. The Maharishi Ayur-Veda system identifies that, on this deeper level, disease is caused by violating the laws of nature.

You've heard the saying, "As you sow, so shall you reap." The Maharishi Ayur-Veda system of health care teaches us how to live in tune with nature so that we sow only seeds that result in health and happiness. Ultimately, this means living in tune with our own inner nature, which is connected to the entire universe.

The Original Mistake

There is a term in the Maharishi Ayur-Veda tradition—*pragya-aparadha*. Literally it means "mistake of the intellect," and it refers to the primary cause of all disease. According to this tradition of health care, on the deepest level there is only one problem, and it's the same for everyone. It is simply forgetting our true nature—our source in pure consciousness and our connectedness to the whole of life. This "forgetting" actually causes fundamental discomfort in the body, and over time creates a chain of events that results in "dis-ease" and eventually symptoms of ill-health.

Fortunately, this is a mistake that is easy to correct, just as turning on the light dispels the darkness. Once we are fully aware, pragya-aparadha is eliminated. And awareness of our true nature—pure

47

consciousness—grows from the inside out through every aspect of the Maharishi Ayur-Veda health program. It is not necessary to think or intellectualize about the process; growth in consciousness is automatic as our health improves and we begin to live the wholeness that we are.

The elimination of pragya-aparadha lies in the realization that "we are already what we want to be." With Maharishi Ayur-Veda health care, day by day, we begin to realize more and more of our full potential. As ama and toxins are flushed out of the system, as we learn how to live in tune with natural law and express more of our inner nature, we free ourselves to become more of what we always were, deep inside—perfectly, radiantly healthy.

Summary

On the most superficial level, disease is caused by an accumulation of toxins and impurities in the body. On a subtler level of functioning, imbalances and violation of natural law are responsible for symptoms of disease. On the subtlest level of all, it is ignorance of our true nature that plants the first seeds of ill-health. Maharishi Ayur-Veda health care provides effective therapies to treat all the root causes of disease.

Part II

Important Therapies of *Maharishi Ayur-Veda* Health Care

Part I provided a basic introduction to the Maharishi Ayur-Veda system of health care. We learned that it offers complete knowledge about life, and that it comes from the oldest tradition known to man. It has been restored to its full value by Maharishi Mahesh Yogi.

The knowledge of this tradition is supremely practical. It has the potential to create perfect health, not only for the individual, but also for society as a whole. Its many therapies are time-tested, natural and very effective.

There are several causes of disease, according to the Maharishi Ayur-Veda system. In the next few chapters, we discuss five Maharishi Ayur-Veda therapies that effectively address all the root causes of disease.

In chapter eight, we describe the Maharishi Transcendental Meditation℠ technique, and its implications for our health. Chapter nine describes how diet can play a significant role in improving health. Powerful, time-tested herbal preparations from the Maharishi Ayur-Veda tradition are the subject of chapter ten. In chapter eleven, we discuss how universal rhythms of life are reflected in our biological rhythms, and how a proper daily routine can be used to balance the functioning of the mind and body. Chapter twelve describes how we can use the larger cycle of the seasons to refresh and rejuvenate ourselves.

These Maharishi Ayur-Veda therapies do more than treat disease. They simultaneously strengthen, nourish and balance the entire mind-body system. Therapies for cure double as measures for prevention. Even while it corrects, this approach always emphasizes the promotion of ideal health and the prevention of further disease.

All Maharishi Ayur-Veda therapies are personalized for your individual needs. The next few chapters describe the different therapies and give general information. But in order for this system to work most effectively for you it is important to see a physician trained in Maharishi Ayur-Veda health care and receive your personalized program for better health. In Part III we will prepare you for this next step.

Chapter Eight

The *Maharishi Transcendental Meditation* Technique

Transcendental Meditation opens the awareness to the infinite reservoir of energy, creativity, and intelligence that lies deep within everyone.

By enlivening this most basic level of life, Transcendental Meditation is that one simple procedure which can raise the life of every individual and every society to its full dignity, in which problems are absent and perfect health, happiness, and a rapid pace of progress are the natural features of life.   —Maharishi Mahesh Yogi

When Maharishi Mahesh Yogi, the founder of the Transcendental Meditation technique, first came to this country in 1959 he was taken aback by news articles describing his meditation. "Non-Medicinal Tranquilizer" was the headline on an article in a San Francisco newspaper, and the piece went on to describe the technique as a way to cure insomnia.

Maharishi was surprised at the article. In India, he said, people turned to meditation to become more fully awake—not to fall asleep! But he knew that no matter why people start the Transcendental Meditation technique, they will get the total effect anyway. The goal they will arrive at will be full enlightenment. And so he decided not to mind the different angles people might take.

Today the TM technique is known for much more than relieving insomnia. Over 500 scientific studies conducted over the past 25 years at more than 200 independent research institutions and universities confirm the wide range of benefits that result from regular daily practice of this simple procedure.[1] To give a few examples in

---

[1] The entire body of research on the Transcendental Meditation technique

53

the field of health alone, studies have found that the TM technique reduces symptoms of bronchial asthma, lowers systolic blood pressure, reduces high blood cholesterol, reverses physiological aging, and dramatically reduces the need for medical care and hospitalization. It also reduces anxiety and tension, reduces the need for caffeine, tobacco, alcohol, and both prescribed and non-prescribed drugs, and improves mental health in general. The technique is perhaps best known, and most often recommended, for its ability to reduce stress.

The regular practice of the Transcendental Meditation technique is one of the most important recommendations that I give to my patients. This is because the TM technique has the most holistic effect. It enlivens pure consciousness, the basis of both the mind and the body, and therefore nourishes all aspects of a person's life simultaneously. It's like watering the root of a tree. All the different parts—trunk, branches, leaves, flowers and fruits—will feel the good effect and flourish.

The patients who take my advice and start the TM technique report not only improvements in their health, but also improvements in every other area of their lives. They notice greater clarity, energy, confidence and creativity, more accomplishment in their daily activity, and increased happiness and fulfillment in their personal relationships—just from the practice of the TM technique.

I recommend the Transcendental Meditation technique even to those patients who are already practicing some other form of meditation or self-development. I tell these patients that I realize they may feel some benefit from what they are doing, and that they don't have to learn the TM technique in order to derive benefits from Maharishi Ayur-Veda health care. But other systems of meditation or self-development all require some effort, either mental

---

has been compiled into six volumes entitled *Scientific Research on Maharishi's Transcendental Meditation and TM-Sidhi Program: Collected Papers*. These books are available through Maharishi University of Management Press, Press Distribution DB 1155, Fairfield, Iowa 52557.

or physical, and this effort will limit the results they can achieve. The TM technique effortlessly allows the mind to experience its own inner nature, pure consciousness, and there are no limits to the benefits one can enjoy. In addition, no other technique has been proven scientifically to produce positive results in all areas of life.

What It Is, What It Is Not

The best news about the TM technique is that it is easy for anyone to do. All it requires is 15–20 minutes twice a day. You sit comfortably in a chair with your eyes closed and practice a simple, natural, effortless procedure that you learn from a qualified teacher[2] over a period of several days. Once you have correctly learned the practice of the TM technique, you can enjoy the benefits for life. Results begin with the very first day of practice, and they continue to grow over time, so it's a wise investment of both time and money.

The Transcendental Meditation technique is not a philosophy, a religion or a way of life. It does not involve concentration, contemplation, or trying to clear your mind of thoughts. It's deeply relaxing and enjoyable—but it's much more than that. The TM technique allows the mind to settle down and enjoy a state of quiet inner alertness, while the body gains a unique state of deep rest that is deeply rejuvenating. This combination of restfulness in the body and alertness in the mind, or "restful alertness," has been shown scientifically to have all the parameters of a fourth major state of consciousness. Unlike deep sleep, unlike dreaming, unlike waking, the TM technique gives the direct experience of unbounded awareness—your innermost self.[3]

---

[2] For information on how to find a qualified teacher of the Transcendental Meditation technique, see chapter nineteen.

[3] See chapter eighteen for a description of the pioneering research on the Transcendental Meditation technique by Dr. Keith Wallace. Dr. Wallace was the first scientist to describe the physical correlates of transcendental consciousness and identify it as a fourth major state of consciousness.

To "transcend" simply means to "go beyond." With the Transcendental Meditation technique you go beyond the surface thinking level of your mind to experience subtler levels of thought, and finally transcend even the subtlest level of thought to experience the source of all thought—a field of pure creative intelligence, pure consciousness. Starting with your very first meditation, the TM technique expands the conscious capacity of the mind, and you begin to live more of your full potential, day by day.

The ultimate benefit of practicing the TM technique is that it raises life to the highest level of human development—to a state traditionally known as "enlightenment." Enlightenment is a big concept that is hard for many people to grasp. But as a physician, I like to think of it in terms of health. Enlightenment to me is nothing more—and nothing less—than invincible health and well-being on all levels of the mind and body.

Maharishi brought the TM technique to the West to eliminate the suffering of mankind in this generation. "The nature of life is bliss" has been his message from the very beginning. "It is not necessary for anyone to suffer." The TM technique is his way to realize that dream. And from my experience, both personally and as a physician, it works.

Summary

The Transcendental Meditation technique gives the direct experience of pure consciousness, which is like watering the "root" of your life. All aspects of your life are simultaneously enriched by the experience of pure consciousness. Because of this, the TM technique is the first and foremost approach of the Maharishi Ayur-Veda system for creating perfect health.

Chapter Nine

Eating Your Way to Health

I purposefully left the word "diet" out of the title for this chapter—even though diet is an important therapy in the Maharishi Ayur-Veda approach. But the word "diet" has come to mean something uncomfortable and unpleasant, something to be endured just for the sake of losing weight or reducing cholesterol.

If your experience with diets has been less than rewarding, you will be happy to know that the first thing I tell my patients about food is that it should be delicious. According to the Maharishi Ayur-Veda system, healthy food is tasty food. It should look good, smell good, and above all taste good.

The Six Tastes

According to this tradition of health care, there are six tastes. A healthy diet will include all six tastes at each main meal. The six tastes are: sweet, sour, salty, pungent, bitter and astringent.

We all know what "sweet" means. But in addition to rich desserts, sugars and other sweeteners, the sweet category includes milk, unsalted butter, rice, wheat, other grains, pasta, breads, and sweet fruits. In the Maharishi Ayur-Veda tradition, all of these foods are considered sweet, although not as obviously sweet as a "spoonful of sugar."

Sour foods include lemons, grapefruit, other tart fruits, vinegar, tomatoes, cheese, yogurt, buttermilk, and other cultured or soured dairy products.

The salty taste comes from the salt that occurs naturally in many foods, as well as by adding salt to our dishes. Anything harvested from the sea, such as seaweed and fish, is usually very salty.

"Pungent" means hot and spicy—as in foods that contain a lot of ginger, cumin, red or green chilies, and black or white pepper.

Some salad ingredients are also naturally hot in taste, such as radishes, watercress, mustard greens and the colorful nasturtiums that add beauty and flavor to a fresh salad.

The bitter taste is found in green leafy vegetables such as kale, spinach, chard and collard greens. Certain spices also have a bitter taste, such as turmeric and fenugreek.

Astringent is the hardest to pin down. Basically, it's the taste that makes your mouth shrink or contract, as often happens with foods that are dry by nature. This taste is found in dried peas and beans, in vegetables such as broccoli, cauliflower, cabbage and potatoes, and in fruits such as apples, pears and pomegranates.

The American diet is heavy on the sweet, sour and salty tastes, and light on the other three. But a balanced diet will include all six tastes, in different proportions according to each person's individual requirements. When you eat all six tastes in the proper proportion for you, you will find that unhealthy cravings fade away, and that naturally you begin to gravitate toward what your body needs most.

A physician trained in Maharishi Ayur-Veda health care will help you determine what's best for you. Some people need more of the satisfying and settling sweet taste; others do best with lots of hot, pungent food that stirs up their physiologies and gets them moving. Sweet and salty, interestingly enough, do not have a bad reputation in the Maharishi Ayur-Veda tradition, when eaten in proper amounts. Sweet is considered to be especially nourishing (like carbohydrates in the Western approach), and salt has a very integrating and grounding effect for those who are "airy" and tend to live in their heads. The only problem comes when a diet is composed of only two or three tastes. "Moderation" is a key word in the Maharishi Ayur-Veda system, and it figures strongly in diet.

Good Taste, Good Health

Taking a good look at the food we eat from the perspective of the six tastes may be new to most people, but in my practice I find that it is a very natural approach. Taste is immediate, and as we all know, extremely satisfying. Taste is, to a large extent, why we eat at all!

It's only recently that people have stopped to analyze their food scientifically and make choices based on nutritional content or calorie count.

Taste has more to do with health than at first we might suspect. On a subtle level, taste is the language nature uses to communicate with the body. Food is nourishing to the body—nourishing not only because it contains vitamins and minerals, proteins and carbohydrates, but because it contains the liveliness of nature's intelligence. This natural intelligence resonates with the body's own intelligence through the direct sensory experience of taste. Eating the right balance of tastes is important because then our inner intelligence is enlivened to the maximum degree.

Food nourishes the body, and it also nourishes the quality of our consciousness. This is due to the intimate connection between the mind and the body—so intimate a connection that it is as if mind and body were woven out of one cloth. Affect one and you directly affect the other.

All of us have noticed at one time or another how the foods we eat affect how we think and feel. Maybe you've felt dull and sluggish after eating too much salt, too much sugar, or too much food in general. Perhaps you've felt fiery and hot-tempered after a meal filled with hot spices. Or are you one of the millions of Americans who needs a morning cup of coffee to wake you up? These are all examples of how the mind is directly affected by what we take into our bodies.

Our society is increasingly aware of the connection between diet and good health. Low-salt, low-fat and high-fiber options are selling like never before. But the connection between diet and consciousness is relatively unknown. Now that knowledge is available through the Maharishi Ayur-Veda system of health care. From this age-old tradition comes complete knowledge about food, including how to determine a proper diet for each person's needs, how to best nourish our minds and bodies, and how to create the highest quality of consciousness through diet.

In the Maharishi Ayur-Veda approach, a proper diet is considered vital for preventing disease and promoting life-long health and longevity. And when it comes to curing disease, diet is considered so important that there is a saying—"Fifty percent of the medicine is proper diet." Similarly, another saying states, "Without proper diet, no medicine will work. With proper diet, no medicine is necessary."

Guidelines for Everyone

In my practice, I always make dietary recommendations. These may be simple and few in number, but there is always some adjustment to the diet that will be helpful for a patient's overall health. And my patients are often amazed at the profound benefits resulting from these simple changes. Just eating more of certain tastes and less of others can make a huge difference in how my patients feel, when those adjustments address their specific needs.

There are some guidelines that apply to everyone. In general, eat a balanced diet that includes all six tastes at least once a day. As much as possible, eat food that is fresh, wholesome and home-cooked. Avoid frozen, canned and preserved foods, fast foods and leftovers. "Nature knows best," so a diet of natural, freshly prepared food, eaten warm, is ideal. According to the Maharishi Ayur-Veda tradition, cooked food is actually more nutritious than raw food for most people, because it is easier to digest and assimilate. It's also better to follow a more vegetarian diet. This does not mean, if you have been eating meat your whole life, that all of a sudden, today, you should stop. Make a slow transition and avoid red meats first. Red meats are heavy and full of fats that are almost impossible to digest. Over time, see if you can limit even poultry and fish.

A vegetarian diet is recommended because it is purer (fewer toxins), more nutritious, and more easily digested. Also, when animals are killed, they are in a state of panic and their systems are flooded with stress hormones that you then consume—along with the nitrites and other chemicals that the meat industry uses to preserve meat for the market.

There is a considerable body of scientific data connecting a vegetarian diet with better health. Vegetarians, for example, are found to have less incidence of chronic degenerative diseases such as heart disease, high blood pressure, obesity, diabetes, osteoporosis and many cancers. In one study, when vegetarians were matched with non-vegetarians and followed for general health, it was found that for every 100 visits made to the doctor by non-vegetarians, vegetarians made only 22 visits, and the numbers were similar for the time spent in hospitals.[1]

The typical vegetarian diet comes closest to meeting the commonly accepted dietary recommendations for healthy eating, because it is low in saturated fats and high in fiber, complex carbohydrates, and fresh fruits and vegetables. For this reason and many others—including taste—consider choosing a more vegetarian diet if you currently favor meat.

Get the Most from Your Food

There are also recommendations for how and when to eat. Not much attention is given to the etiquette of eating anymore, and many people make a habit of eating on the run, in their cars, or at their desks. But in the Maharishi Ayur-Veda system, how you eat is just as important as what you eat.

To maximize the intelligence you receive from your food, it's important to take the time to really taste it. Tasting your food alerts the body to what is coming, and actually primes your digestive system to do its job properly and completely. When you pay attention to your food, you are also more likely to eat the proper amount and stop when you feel full.

Give full attention to your food and really enjoy it. Resist the temptation to listen to music, read the morning paper or turn on the evening news. Have your meals in a settled environment and always

---

[1] Dickerson, J., and J. Davies. "Consequences for Health of a Vegetarian Diet." Postdoctoral thesis, University of Surrey, England, 1986.

61

sit to eat. Don't bring work, important decisions, bad moods or arguments to the table.

Eat at regular times every day. That way, the body becomes habituated to periods of rest and activity, and brings its full power to the job at hand. It's also ideal to eat your main meal at midday, if possible, because that is when your digestive powers are naturally at their peak. If you eat at night, it should be early and light.

Avoid snacking. The body doesn't know what to do with snacks because it is busy digesting the previous meal. Digestion is bound to be poor and incomplete when you are always reaching for snacks.

All of these guidelines may seem like common sense—and they are. But if you make them a habit in your life, they can make a big difference in how well your body digests what you give it, and how much nourishment you receive. They also make a big difference in how much enjoyment you receive from your food.

Enjoying food is one of life's simple pleasures. When it comes to diet and Maharishi Ayur-Veda health care, the big picture is clear. Eat a variety of food, make it appealing and tasty, and take the time to really enjoy it. Food is more than calories and portion sizes—it is nature's gift. The attention you give to your diet will come back to you many times over in the form of increased vitality, greater well-being, and a purer, more enlightened consciousness.

Summary

Food is nourishing because it contains the intelligence of nature, which enlivens body, mind and consciousness. The Maharishi Ayur-Veda system of health care provides complete knowledge about diet to maximize the natural intelligence we can receive from our food.

Chapter Ten

Nature's Pharmacy

The names sound like poetry. "Heart-leaved moonseed," "East Indian globe thistle," "Himalayan silver fir," "Bengal quince," "elephant creeper," "cashmere bark," "trumpet flower."

There are others—perhaps not quite so poetic!—"spreading hogweed," "giant potato," "shoe flower." Many have never been translated because there is no English equivalent—"teramnus labialis," "eragrostis cynosuroides."

These are just a few of the thousands of herbal ingredients that go into the time-tested formulas of the Maharishi Ayur-Veda tradition.

Not all are unfamiliar. Many of the ingredients would feel right at home on your kitchen shelf. Cumin, cinnamon, saffron, black pepper, raisins and honey are just a few examples.

Maharishi Ayur-Veda herbal formulas are the most ancient in the world. Prepared precisely according to tradition, they usually contain mixtures of many different herbs—sometimes as many as forty or fifty.

Synergistic Effects

The exact combination of herbs is important. There is a saying— "The whole is more than the sum of its parts"—and it applies here. The whole of all the herbal ingredients together is much more powerful and balancing than the sum of the individual parts. This combined effect is like a kind of advanced synergy to help strengthen the entire mind-body system.

The last chapter described how the foods we eat contain the liveliness of nature's intelligence and how, with a proper diet, we can use this intelligence to nourish the body. With herbs this natural intelligence is even more concentrated, more powerful—but the principle is the same. Like resonates with like, and the laws of nature found in herbs can be used very effectively to resonate with the body's own inner intelligence and correct any slight mistake or imbalance.

Each herb in a given formula contains a different value of nature's intelligence. And each herb has an important role to play, somewhat the way each instrument in a symphony orchestra makes an important contribution to the music being performed. Some herbs target problem areas of the body. Other herbs are included to make sure the target herbs are properly assimilated and digested. Still others nourish the entire mind-body system while the problem is being corrected, or are included just to provide balancing effects.

Western medicine specializes in isolating "active ingredients." This is partly because of the limitations of the scientific laboratory method, which tests only one thing at a time under tightly controlled conditions. But the use of isolated, so-called "active" ingredients in pharmaceutical drugs often results in harmful side effects.

Most large pharmaceutical companies are eager to research and explore the uses of traditional plants. Examples of modern drugs that are derived from natural sources include aspirin (from willow bark), digitalis (from foxglove), morphine (from poppy), and quinine (from the bark of a swamp plant that flourishes in malarial areas). But modern science does not appreciate the real dangers of isolating powerful ingredients, nor does it understand how important it is to combine ingredients to minimize side effects. The Maharishi Ayur-Veda tradition provides exactly what is needed—a systematic theoretical understanding of how herbs interact and how to combine them to create an overall nourishing effect. Moreover, Maharishi Ayur-Veda herbal formulas are supported by thousands of years of actual clinical experience, which provides an accumulated wisdom in the practical application of herbs that cannot be duplicated in any modern scientific laboratory.

Maharishi Ayur-Veda herbal supplements strengthen, nourish and balance the entire system. Each ingredient in a formula is considered "active"—that is, a necessary part of the whole—and is carefully balanced by other ingredients to ensure that your path to better health is comfortable and secure.

The Value of Tradition

Just as important as the actual ingredients is the way they are prepared. According to the Maharishi Ayur-Veda system, the only way to prepare medicinal herbs is the traditional way—just as described in the age-old texts. Only with traditional processing methods can you be assured of getting the full benefits.

Shortcuts won't do. Raising the temperature, for example, may reduce processing time, but it also destroys the subtle nutritive value of delicate herbs and spices. Sometimes proper preparation calls for many hundreds of steps, and each one is considered vital. In addition, all Maharishi Ayur-Veda herbal preparations are thoroughly tested for purity, potency and your safety as a consumer.

Formulas from the Maharishi Ayur-Veda tradition were restored to authenticity by the greatest exponents of Ayur-Veda, who came together under the guidance and inspiration of Maharishi Mahesh Yogi. These physicians are: Dr. V.M. Dwivedi, a great leader in the science of special herbal formulas called *rasayanas*; Dr. B.D. Triguna, the greatest living expert in the science of pulse diagnosis; and Dr. Balaraj Maharshi, the world's foremost expert in the identification and application of medicinal plants.

Herbs for Every Need

Maharishi Ayur-Veda herbal formulas are of two kinds. One class is primarily for overall nourishment and revitalization. These formulas, called rasayanas, have as their purpose the prevention of disease and the promotion of ideal health.

The "king" of rasayanas is the Maharishi Amrit Kalash formula ("Amrit" for short), and I recommend this for almost everyone. According to the tradition, Amrit promotes *bala,* or vital energy. It also strengthens the immune system and refines the functioning of the physiology to support the experience of higher states of consciousness. Scientific studies show that Amrit fights damaging free radicals 1,000 times more effectively than any other antioxidant (see chapter seven).

There are hundreds of other rasayanas described in the ancient texts: rasayanas for women, for men, for the mind, the heart, the liver, the skin, and every other major organ and system in the body. I recommend these rasayanas when needed, depending on a patient's individual situation.

The other class of Maharishi Ayur-Veda herbal formulations is taken to correct specific imbalances which may be detected in a particular patient. These preparations address underlying problems, the root cause of a patient's complaint. By following a complete Maharishi Ayur-Veda program, including the use of herbs, many of my patients see improvement within the first few weeks. Of course, some problems are more difficult to address. Maharishi Ayur-Veda herbal preparations are usually taken for three to six months, but in some cases I recommend that they be taken longer.

Unlike many over-the-counter and prescription drugs, Maharishi Ayur-Veda herbs do not simply mask symptoms. Nor do they interfere with the normal functioning of the body or try to supply something that is not already there. They work with the body and its own inner intelligence to correct the situation from within. It's as if the body needed reminding how to take care of itself in the most efficient way. Maharishi Ayur-Veda herbal remedies act as a gentle reminder and enliven natural pathways of intelligence so that the system is again self-sufficient.

As a physician, it is a joy to have as my resource the most extensive pharmacopoeia on earth. But more than that, from the Maharishi Ayur-Veda tradition I have the knowledge of how to apply this powerful herbal technology to benefit my patients. It is truly gratifying to witness the profound effects of Maharishi Ayur-Veda herbal formulas.

Stories about the power of herbs are found in traditional cultures all over the world. One tale in particular that I remember from my own childhood comes from the *Ramayana*. It is the story of Hanuman rescuing the fallen army with healing herbs from the Himalayas.

Hanuman is known as the "monkey god" in India and is the son of the wind god. When Rama's army was lying wounded and dying on the battlefield, Hanuman was dispatched to the peaks of the Himalayas to fetch celestial healing herbs. The herbs he was sent to find had the power to restore vitality, heal all wounds, join severed limbs, mend broken bones, and bring the dead back to life. Such was Hanuman's power that when he reached the Himalayas he uprooted an entire mountain peak and flew with it back to the army's aid. The story says that the soldiers were healed on the spot simply by inhaling the fragrance of the powerful herbs. Those who were unconscious leapt to their feet, wounds were healed all at once, pain vanished in an instant.

I have not seen miracles as dramatic as this, but I have often thought that the Maharishi Ayur-Veda herbs I use in my daily practice are related to those celestial herbs from the *Ramayana*. The miracles I see are quiet ones, but they are miracles nonetheless. Maharishi Ayur-Veda herbs play a key role as part of a complete Maharishi Ayur-Veda program to create better health.

Summary

The knowledge of how to use herbs to create better health is part of the age-old Maharishi Ayur-Veda tradition. Maharishi Ayur-Veda herbal formulas enliven the body's inner intelligence and help the body regain its own natural state of balance.

Chapter Eleven

Nature's Clock

Have you ever wondered how the morning cock knows when to crow? Or how the birds, calling to each other in the twilight, know when it's time to go to bed?

Nature loves rhythms. And everywhere in nature, you'll see living things following natural rhythms, as easily and effortlessly as flowers unfolding in sunshine. There's no partying past bedtime, or sleeping in late. There's no checking watches, or marking the calendar. Birds never forget to migrate; fish never decide they'll skip school. Nature's laws are absolute—and they are all-nourishing.

It's only human beings who break the rules. Living in crowded urban areas, with electric lights that outshine the stars, it's easy to forget that we're a part of nature too. But the laws of nature that govern the universe are the very same laws that govern our minds and bodies.

The timeless knowledge of the Maharishi Ayur-Veda tradition is like a wise teacher reminding us who we really are and what it means to live naturally. The knowledge is simple, and yet very profound. As the verse from ancient Vedic literature says, "As is the atom, so is the universe; as is the body, so is the cosmic body."

One of the most practical aspects of the Maharishi Ayur-Veda approach is the knowledge of how to follow an ideal daily routine. According to this system of health care, following a good routine—day in and day out—is one of the most powerful things we can do to prevent disease and create ideal health. By following a good routine we actually synchronize our internal biological rhythms with the universal rhythms of nature. Western science is just beginning to understand the significance of biological rhythms, but this sophisticated knowledge has been part of the Maharishi Ayur-Veda tradition from the beginning.

The Maharishi Ayur-Veda system of health care provides not only guidelines for what to do when, but also profound knowledge about the laws of nature that operate at different times of the day and night. These laws of nature influence us in very direct ways, and it's good to be aware of them. When we understand how we are being influenced by our environment, then we can "go with the flow" of nature's intelligence. Life becomes easier and we encounter less resistance.

Once you experience the patterns of normal living for yourself— patterns that nature always intended for us to live—I think you'll understand what it means to feel the "support of natural law." Living in tune with nature is like swimming downstream—it's effortless. Once the rhythm is established, you can relax and enjoy the scenery. Nature does all the work for you, and delivers you quickly and safely to your goal.

Early to Bed, Early to Rise

As you might imagine, it's best to wake up early—"with the birds." In the early dawn hours, there is a liveliness in nature that is not available at any other time of the day. When you wake up early, you take advantage of that liveliness and carry it into the day with you.

The trick to waking up early—and naturally, too, without using an alarm clock—is to go to bed early. Going to bed between nine and ten o'clock is ideal. You'll find that it's actually easier to fall asleep when you go to bed early, and that your sleep is deeper and more refreshing.

Morning Massage

A highlight of the Maharishi Ayur-Veda morning routine is a warm-oil massage (*abhyanga*) before you shower or bathe in the morning. Giving yourself a morning massage is a great way to wake up (much better than reaching for a cup of coffee!), and it also improves circulation, tones muscles, increases flexibility in tissues and joints, removes toxins, rejuvenates the skin, and balances the entire physiology. Moreover, it helps you start the day with a relaxed attitude, which is very beneficial for your overall health. People who approach the day as a race against time do not have the best chance of creating perfect health.

Self-massage feels good—and that's just the beginning of the story. The skin contains thousands of nerves that are connected to every part of the body, inside and out. Science also recognizes that the skin is a major producer of endocrine hormones. So when we massage the skin we actually enhance two master systems of the body—the nervous system and the endocrine system. Using sesame oil for your massage is also recommended because sesame oil is gently warming and strengthens immunity.

Patients who do abhyanga regularly report that they feel the benefits all day long. They feel smoother in activity, less overshadowed by events, emotionally more stable. Patients who have dry, rough skin and patients who tend to have cold hands and feet are especially appreciative of the warm, lubricating effects of morning oil massage.

Doing abhyanga is a delightful way to give yourself nourishing attention. You deserve the pampering! And the effects are deep and far-reaching. By using the sense of touch, with your innocent attention on the body as you perform the massage, you actually integrate the lively value of your awareness into the concrete matter of the body. As with all Maharishi Ayur-Veda therapies, the ultimate accomplishment is development of consciousness—which improves your health as a whole.

It takes only a few minutes every morning to perform abhyanga. A physician trained in Maharishi Ayur-Veda health care can teach you the exact procedure.

What about Exercise?

My patients often ask about the need for exercise, and what the Maharishi Ayur-Veda approach has to offer. Exercise is important, but recommendations are highly individual, based on each person's

71

situation and needs. There are a few guidelines, however, that apply to everyone.

Proper exercise, according to the ancient texts of Ayur-Veda, gives the body lightness. It gives you energy and vitality, increases your capacity for work, helps to release stress and toxins from the system, increases your stamina and endurance, firms the muscles, and stimulates the digestion. Everything works better and feels better when you exercise properly.

What is proper exercise? Not too much, for one thing. Here in the West there is almost a mania for pushing the body to its limits. According to the Maharishi Ayur-Veda tradition, exercise should give you more energy than it takes. You should feel exhilarated and refreshed after you exercise, not exhausted, sweaty and tired. So the general guideline is to exercise up to only half your capacity. That means if you can run six miles, run only three. If you can swim twenty laps, go for ten. These lower limits actually make exercise more efficient, because you're not giving the body repair work to do afterwards, and your cardiovascular system can return to normal much faster. Another way to tell that you've had enough is to go until you feel yourself starting to sweat, or until you start to breathe heavily. These are nature's signs that you are at the right limit.

Walking is an exercise that comes close to being ideal for everyone. A brisk walk for half an hour a day is highly recommended in the Maharishi Ayur-Veda tradition. If you are of slight build and have little stamina, set a leisurely pace for yourself. If you are strong, solid and sometimes feel sluggish, try walking faster. You will naturally feel stimulated and lighter by the end of your walk.

Yoga *asanas* (postures) are also highly recommended for almost everyone because they increase circulation, improve mind-body coordination, and develop both flexibility and strength. You can learn specialized sets of asanas by taking courses at your local Maharishi Ayur-Veda University or School (see chapter nineteen for details). One classic set of twelve postures, called *Surya Namaskara*, systematically enlivens all the major systems of the body, and it takes only a few minutes to do. In the Maharishi Ayur-Veda approach, the idea is to create balance, not put on a perfect performance, so don't worry about how you look or how close you come to the "ideal position." Whatever you achieve is right for you and accomplishes the goal.

Other tips: do your exercise in the morning, after the sun is up. This is when the physiology is naturally strongest and most vital. It's the time when all of nature is busily engaged in activity, and it's the best time for you to be active too.

When you exercise, do not distract the mind by listening to music, watching TV, or carrying on a conversation. Give your full attention to your body and enjoy yourself. Distracting the mind during exercise actually destroys the intimate connection between the mind and body. When you are "out of touch" with your body, it's easy to go too far or injure yourself unknowingly.

Nature has given us a great gift in the mind-body connection. When you become attuned to your body through proper exercise you begin to appreciate that your body is not just "there." It is very intimately yourself, clothed in matter. Getting back in touch with your physical self through exercise can be a very delightful experience, especially for those who have given up on exercise and are virtual strangers to their bodies.

Time for Food

Food is a central part of everyone's daily routine, and in this respect Maharishi Ayur-Veda health care has much to offer. First of all, it is important to eat food that is right for you and your needs. Your physician will help you plan an ideal diet.

We have already written about eating a proper, balanced diet that includes all six tastes (see chapter nine). We have also discussed giving yourself the best chance to digest your food properly and completely. This means eating in a settled way, and allowing enough time between meals for thorough digestion.

There is another important food guideline that applies to all. If possible, it's best to eat your largest meal at midday. This is because the sun is at its peak at noon, and your digestive "fire" is also naturally at its peak. When you eat at noon, you are working with nature, and your food will be digested more quickly and completely. At dawn and sunset, there is little digestive fire in the stomach—just as there is not much heat in the day. Therefore, a light breakfast and a light supper are recommended in the Maharishi Ayur-Veda tradition.

So forget the old saying, "Eat breakfast like a king"! Eat a light breakfast if you like. But save your appetite for a hearty noontime lunch.

Likewise, the later you eat, the lighter you should eat. In the evening, avoid heavy foods such as meat, cheeses and other cultured foods completely, because they are hard to digest even under the best of conditions.

Some of my patients complain to me that it is impossible to eat their main meal at midday due to pressures at home or at work. I tell them, you can arrange it if you want to! It only requires some creativity and a little determination. I am amazed at the ingenuity my patients display in managing their daily routines. And they come back and tell me that it's worth the effort, that they never felt better in their lives.

Moderation in All Things

Most people spend many hours a day working to earn a living. So it would be neglectful to devote an entire chapter to daily routine without mentioning work. What does Maharishi Ayur-Veda health care have to offer in this respect?

First of all, it is important to like your work. Job satisfaction is one of the factors most associated with good health. If your work is right for you, you will feel nourished and energized at the end of the day, not tired or burned out. It's also important to create a positive work environment. Obviously, a noisy or smoke-filled environment does not contribute to good health. But on a subtler level, an environment filled with negativity, stress, back-biting and bickering will also eat away at your health and happiness. See if you can find work that you really enjoy, and put some attention on structuring a work environment that is pleasant and supportive.[1]

"Moderation in all things" is our motto. Work should never overshadow other areas of life that are just as important. Take time to play. Take time to enjoy your family. Take time for the simple joys of life. Enjoy the beauties of nature. Live a balanced life—enough of everything.

Regularity is also a key to the Maharishi Ayur-Veda daily routine. Regularity of habits, more than anything, helps to create balance. Regularity of rest, regularity of exercise, regularity of mealtimes, regularity in work hours—regularity helps. Even on weekends, when you may be tempted to stay up late and sleep in, or break the routine in some other way (pizza at midnight!), remember that life thrives on regularity. Once you experience how consistently good you can feel when you honor the flow of an ideal daily routine, in accord with the rhythms of nature, you'll never look back at the so-called "pleasures of life."

Winding Down

Have we reached the end of the day? Remember your ten o'clock bedtime! Even earlier is better. Everything in nature winds down with the setting of the sun, and you should too. Even if you cannot fall asleep when you get into bed, that's fine. Lie there comfortably, not minding. You are still getting the rest and rejuvenation that you need. Most of my patients find that it takes just a few nights to adjust, and that it's actually easier to fall asleep the earlier they go to bed.

Nature is like one big clock, chiming the hours if we know how to listen. The Maharishi Ayur-Veda tradition reminds us that we are

---

[1] Many research studies on the Transcendental Meditation technique have shown that those practicing the TM technique enjoy increased job satisfaction, increased efficiency and productivity, improved relations with coworkers, and better mental and physical health. For more information, see chapter eight and chapter eighteen.

a part of nature, and that if we obey her rules we will enjoy the rewards. For ideal health, listen to Mother Nature. Follow her example and establish a daily routine that will nourish life and bring it to fulfillment.

Summary

Using behavior to balance the mind and body can be a powerful way to create better health. The Maharishi Ayur-Veda system of health care provides complete knowledge about universal rhythms of life that are reflected in our biological rhythms, and gives guidelines for how to work with nature in structuring an ideal daily routine.

Chapter Twelve

Seasonal Rejuvenation

There was a time when, in every household, "spring" meant "housecleaning." With vigor and determination, the women of the house would turn everything inside out. Curtains would come down, to be laundered and pressed fresh. Furniture would be moved away from walls, and the accumulated dirt scrubbed away. Rugs would be hung outside, and beaten until no more dust flew. Cabinets would be emptied and washed, windows thrown open, and the whole house aired. Finally, to the children's delight, it was time to put away scratchy winter woolens and bring out the light cottons of spring and summer.

On the farm, spring meant checking the machinery and farm tools, oiling and sharpening them for the coming season. The land was cleared, soil prepared and plans finalized. Weather was followed closely, for farmers in every age have always needed to work hand in hand with nature to produce a crop.

Nature has its own way of "cleaning house" and preparing for springtime. With the warmth of longer days comes the rush of water through every rivulet as melting snow finds its way to the ocean. Floods and seasonal wetlands are nature's way of sweeping away the debris of winter, fertilizing the land for a summertime of growth, and depositing upstream soil downstream, creating new beaches for different species to live and thrive. The entire ecosystem is cleansed and enriched by nature's springtime bath.

Is there anything we can do, inside and out, to cleanse and rejuvenate ourselves in a similar way? Most of us feel the itchiness of spring's "fever," but don't quite know what to do about it. Maybe it's nature's signal that it's time to participate in a bigger cycle— bigger than our daily and monthly cycles and routines. Maybe it's time to break the routine with a bigger pattern of life—the cycle of the seasons.

Maharishi Ayur-Veda health care has the perfect cure for spring fever. It's called the Maharishi Rejuvenation℠ program and what it does is gently "houseclean" our bodies from the inside out. It sweeps away accumulated debris, and freshens and sharpens our entire system for another season of efficient functioning.

The Maharishi Rejuvenation program is actually a combination of treatments administered over a period of a few days at regional Maharishi Ayur-Veda Medical Centers. It is one of the most powerful therapies for creating life-long health, and is therefore often recommended by physicians trained in the Maharishi Ayur-Veda approach.

Change of Season, Change of Style

It's natural to adjust to the coming of a new season. We automatically change our wardrobe, for example, to reflect changes in the temperature—shedding layers in the spring, and putting them back on in the fall. In the summer, it's natural to eat more of the sweet fresh fruits and vegetables that are available locally, whereas winter finds us choosing hot soups and hearty stews. Likewise, we look for ways to enjoy the great outdoors in spring and summer, but busy ourselves with indoor projects in the dark of winter. These are natural adjustments to our environment, and we usually don't think twice about them.

What the Maharishi Ayur-Veda tradition adds is the knowledge of how to adjust on a deeper level. According to this tradition, each new season brings a fundamental change in the underlying laws of nature, and it's important for us to know how to adapt, in order to keep ourselves fit and healthy. How many of us almost expect to catch the flu as winter approaches, or a nasty cold come springtime? We take seasonal ailments for granted, but they are nature's signs that we have not taken proper precautions to adapt to fundamental changes in nature.

According to the Maharishi Ayur-Veda system, it's important to "start fresh" with the beginning of each new season. For example, by the end of winter, the rough, dry, cold and windy qualities of winter tend to accumulate in our systems, causing subtle imbalances that need to be corrected. Likewise, by the end of summer, the unrelenting heat outside has us fired up inside, creating additional wear and tear. Seasonal rejuvenation purifies the system of any accumulated effects due to climate and environment, balances the system to work in harmony with nature, and gives us the fresh start we need to face a new season in good health.

Seasonal rejuvenation also removes toxins that have accumulated in the system due to poor diet and digestion, and removes deep-seated fatigue that comes from an improper daily routine. The procedures of seasonal rejuvenation actually open up the body's channels, sweep away obstructions, and give the entire system the experience of truly "normal" functioning.

Is it any surprise that patients who choose seasonal rejuvenation feel like they shed years in just a matter of days? In fact, research on seasonal rejuvenation indicates that it is a very powerful way to increase biological youthfulness and improve overall well-being.

In one study, subjects participating in a one-week seasonal rejuvenation program improved significantly in a variety of health parameters, including energy and vitality, strength and stamina, appetite and digestion, and state of mind and emotions.[1] Another study showed significant declines in unhealthy emotional states such as anxiety, depression, fatigue and confusion.[2] (See chapter eighteen.)

Seasonal rejuvenation also produces profound effects on the cellular level. In one study it was found that 3–5 days of seasonal rejuvenation reduced serum lipid peroxide levels while it increased vasoactive intestinal peptide and HDL or "good" cholesterol.

---

[1] *The Journal of Social Behavior and Personality* 5 (1990): 1–27.

[2] R.H. Schneider, K. Cavanaugh, S. Rothenberg, R. Averbach, R.K. Wallace. "Improvements in Health with the Maharishi Ayur-Veda Prevention Program." Paper presented at the International College of Psychosomatic Medicine, Eighth World Congress, Chicago, Illinois, September 1985.

At the same time, the subjects showed a lessening of anxiety and reduced diastolic blood pressure. All of these results indicate that seasonal rejuvenation reduces cardiovascular risk factors.[3]

The Ultimate Refreshment

As with all Maharishi Ayur-Veda therapies, seasonal rejuvenation is personalized for your individual health needs. Treatment usually begins with a gentle internal cleansing program that you do yourself (as per your physician's instructions) at home. It involves taking a special herb or oil (as prescribed) on four or more consecutive days. This is followed by a gentle laxative treatment on the evening of the fourth day. This initial step, called "home preparation," is a valuable therapy in and of itself, and begins the process of purification.

The "in-house" portion of the treatment is administered only at licensed Maharishi Ayur-Veda Medical Centers—and it comes close to matching most people's idea of heaven! The program is designed first and foremost to provide deep rest and relaxation so that the body is free to purify itself on fundamental levels. When you check in for seasonal rejuvenation, you "check out" of your life as usual, leaving worries and cares behind you. Then, in a safe and comfortable environment, you receive personalized treatments that systematically stimulate the circulation, open the channels of the body, loosen old deposits of toxins, and gently eliminate them from the body.

The program often includes heat treatments such as herbalized full-body steam baths or the application of warm herbalized oils and pastes. Variations on treatments are innumerable, because each person's needs are unique. Your program is tailored to meet your needs. For those suffering from serious or chronic diseases there are special additional therapies.

All of the treatments are designed exactly as specified in the age-old texts. Nothing is improvised; nothing is by chance. This is your guarantee of complete safety, and your assurance that you will

---

[3] *The Journal of Research and Education in Indian Medicine* 12 (1993): 3–13.

get the full benefits. Like all Maharishi Ayur-Veda therapies, seasonal rejuvenation has passed the test of time, and it works because it normalizes the body on deeper, more profound levels of its functioning.

Your program is supervised by a doctor trained in Maharishi Ayur-Veda health care, and administered by a well-trained staff devoted to serving your every need. The program includes comfortable accommodations, nourishing meals, and ample opportunities to learn more about the Maharishi Ayur-Veda approach and how to create better health. You always leave the center with a complete home preventive program—as well as a fresh "new" physiology to face the challenges of the coming months.[4]

Many of my patients can't wait for another season to pass so they can go for seasonal treatment. Seasonal rejuvenation is like basking in the lap of luxury, like being soothed and pampered, revitalized and refreshed, all at the same time. It's the ultimate vacation, the ultimate self-indulgence.

And just think—it's good for your health!

Summary

The Maharishi Rejuvenation program fine-tunes the system to adapt to laws of nature that change from season to season. By eliminating accumulated impurities and correcting imbalances that have built up over time, it effectively refreshes the system and prepares it for another season of proper functioning.

---

[4] Seasonal rejuvenation treatments are often available on an out-patient basis for those who live within easy commuting distance of a Maharishi Ayur-Veda Medical Center.

Part III

Working with a Physician Trained in *Maharishi Ayur-Veda* Health Care

In Part II we discussed five therapies that are frequently recommended by physicians practicing Maharishi Ayur-Veda health care. There are many different therapies, but these few should give a feeling for the complete scope of this age-old system.

The advantage of the Maharishi Ayur-Veda system of health care is that it uses every possible means to create and maintain health. Some of the approaches work through the mind (such as the Transcendental Meditation technique); some work through the body (such as diet). Other approaches work with our behavior and daily activity, or emphasize our interaction with the environment. Wherever there is a way to enliven the inner intelligence of our minds and bodies, Maharishi Ayur-Veda health care has something to offer. Each approach works effectively by itself, and each works powerfully in conjunction with others. In fact, all of the approaches complement and support each other to multiply the overall effect—the whole is more than the sum of its parts.

In this next part, we will discuss the specialized knowledge available from physicians trained in Maharishi Ayur-Veda health care and what you might expect if you decide to try this approach for yourself. Chapter thirteen presents basic information about the three fundamental organizing principles of nature (called Vata, Pitta and Kapha), and how these principles operate in your mind and body. This information is central to understanding how Maharishi Ayur-Veda health care applies to your individual situation.

In chapter fourteen we describe a powerful technique used by every physician trained in this system—the technique of pulse diagnosis. Pulse diagnosis is more than checking the vitality of the cardiovascular system or counting beats per minute; it provides detailed information on imbalances in Vata, Pitta and Kapha that exist anywhere in the body. It is one of the "secrets" that makes Maharishi Ayur-Veda health care so effective in the prevention and treatment of disease.

In chapter fifteen we discuss your relationship with your doctor and how to make it work most effectively for you. We also discuss what you might expect from your treatment over time.

Nothing in a book can replace the personalized information that you receive from your doctor, but we can give you enough general information to prepare you, and "set the stage" for what might be the greatest adventure of your life. Are you ready?

Chapter Thirteen

Vata, Pitta and Kapha

At first glance they mean nothing. They are just words without association. But as you become familiar with the concepts of Vata, Pitta and Kapha, and apply them to your everyday life, I think you will agree that this specialized knowledge from the Maharishi Ayur-Veda tradition provides a valuable key to unlock mysteries in yourself and the world around you.

Vata, Pitta and Kapha are the three main organizing principles of nature. Each principle has qualities by which it can be recognized. Vata is moving, quick, light, clear, cold, subtle, brittle, rough and dry. Pitta is hot, sharp, liquid, pungent, acidic and slightly oily. Kapha is heavy, slow, steady, stable, solid, sweet, cold, sticky, unctuous, soft and dull.

If you are confused already, don't worry! Things will become clear as we go along. For now, think of Vata, Pitta and Kapha as a kind of master theoretical framework that will help you learn more about life.

Let's start by applying Vata, Pitta and Kapha to ourselves and give a few examples. In the body, Vata, Pitta and Kapha govern the flow of the body's inner intelligence. They regulate all the different functions of our minds as well as our bodies.

Vata, Pitta and Kapha at Work

Vata is the only moving principle, so wherever you see movement, you see Vata in operation. Vata governs respiration, circulation, elimination, and neuromuscular activity. It also governs the quick and lively activity of our minds and five senses.

In many ways, Vata is "boss." Because it is the only principle that moves, it leads the other two principles. They depend on Vata to get their respective jobs done. When Vata is in balance and does its work well, that helps Pitta and Kapha. If there is a problem with Vata, then it's easy for Pitta and Kapha to develop problems too.

Pitta is the only hot principle. It manages digestion and metabolism, keeps bodily heat in balance, and regulates hunger and thirst. Pitta is also the governing principle behind sharp decision-making, creative intelligence, and warm feelings of joy and contentment.

Kapha is cold like the Vata principle, but the coldness of Kapha is heavy and wet, not light and dry like Vata. Kapha is responsible for solid body structure and fluid balance. It gives potency, solidity and strength to the body, and keeps all joints smooth and well-lubricated. Kapha is also found in a sweet, steady and affectionate heart, and is the principle supporting forgiveness, generosity and courage.

When you consult a physician trained in Maharishi Ayur-Veda health care, the first thing that he or she will assess is how well Vata, Pitta and Kapha are doing their jobs. Are they strong and functioning properly? Are they in their right places and minding their own business? What is the degree of balance or imbalance?

If your physician detects any imbalances, then they will need to be addressed. Such imbalances, if untended, eventually result in symptoms of discomfort and disease.

If you suffer already from symptoms of disease, then your doctor will determine what fundamental imbalances in the functioning of Vata, Pitta and Kapha are responsible. All of the recommendations that you receive from your doctor are designed to correct these fundamental imbalances and reestablish harmony in the mind and body.

How does your doctor know what needs attention? He will take into account many factors gathered from talking to you and observing you. He will ask basic questions about your health, your digestion, your sleep, your level of energy, your lifestyle and your choice of foods. Most importantly, he will use a technique called Maharishi Ayur-Veda pulse diagnosis to determine the specific imbalances which may be present in your physiology. Your pulse also gives the doctor additional and detailed information about how well Vata, Pitta and Kapha are functioning. (We will describe more about pulse diagnosis in chapter fourteen.)

How They Work Together

Vata, Pitta and Kapha are never found in isolation. Everyone has all three principles, always working together. Ideally, Vata, Pitta and Kapha function in perfect balance. But often, our habits of living and eating contribute to the development of certain imbalances.

Let's take an example. Bonnie is in her forties. She is quick-moving and vivacious. She is passionate about her work, which involves working with people and computers. She loves to travel, and her work often takes her on business trips both in this country and abroad. She gets up early, works long hours, and often skips lunch to fit in an hour of exercise.

Bonnie works hard, and she plays hard. Her weekends are full of varied and interesting activities with her husband and friends— bike trips, art and antique shopping, dinners out. Often she is absorbed in a big home improvement project such as planting a new garden or redecorating, and she does most of the work herself.

Bonnie's home is her anchor. She lives in the same town where she grew up, and has lived in the same house with her husband for over twenty years. Even though her commute to work takes two hours each day, she would never consider moving.

Bonnie's health is good in general, but she suffers from anxiety over situations at work, and will often come down with a cold or the flu after an extended business trip. She puts a lot of pressure on herself to be perfect, and can be very critical and demanding of herself as well as others. She also feels a lot of anger and finds it hard to let go of grievances.

Even from this brief profile, we can see all three principles at work in Bonnie's mind and body. She is lively, enthusiastic, and feels excited about her work and life in general. These characteristics reflect the quick and moving qualities of Vata.

The Pitta principle can be seen in the intensity of her commitment to work, family and friends, in her strong competitive spirit and inner drive to excel, and in how well she organizes and manages her busy life. These are all Pitta characteristics, reflecting the warm, sharp qualities of Pitta.

The Kapha principle can be seen in her rootedness to home, in the stability of her relationships, and, physically, in her beautiful soft skin, strong facial features, and thick dark hair. These characteristics reflect the heavy, solid, steady and soft qualities of Kapha.

We can also see some symptoms of imbalance in Bonnie. Anxiety is usually associated with a Vata imbalance, anger and resentment with a Pitta imbalance. Moreover, her tendency to get sick after traveling shows that her immune system is weak, which usually means that Kapha needs strengthening.

I would give Bonnie a Maharishi Ayur-Veda program that helps to balance all three principles. For example, I would suggest that Bonnie use her lunch hour to eat rather than exercise, and that she work out in the mornings or early evenings instead. Eating a big lunch would help balance Vata because Vata thrives on regularity. Eating at the same time every day stabilizes and grounds the Vata principle, which is light and airy by nature. A big midday meal would also help balance Pitta because Pitta, being hot and fiery by nature, needs substantial fuel to govern itself properly. And it would simultaneously balance Kapha, because Bonnie would get the nourishment she needs to maintain her strength. Eating at midday, Bonnie would also have enough time to digest her food completely and efficiently, which helps all three principles.

Just this one recommendation can make a huge difference in how Bonnie feels. As her Vata comes more into balance, she will find that she is less anxious and more settled inside, no matter what the outside circumstances. As her Pitta comes more into balance and her body's needs are taken care of, she will find that she is happier and more contented on a daily basis. And as her Kapha comes more into balance, she will find that her energy level is high and her immune system strong, even when she is faced with unusual demands.

Of course, in a Maharishi Ayur-Veda consultation, Bonnie would also receive personalized recommendations for what foods to eat, what kind of exercise to do, and what herbs to take to strengthen her physiology and correct imbalances—as well as other Maharishi Ayur-Veda therapies. She would receive a complete Maharishi Ayur-Veda program that would address all her needs and set her on a sure course for successful preventive health care.

Bonnie is just one example of how Vata, Pitta and Kapha can work together. Not everyone is like Bonnie. Bonnie leads an active life, and in many ways, it is the non-stop pace of her high-energy lifestyle that has led to certain imbalances. In contrast, we all know people who lead very sedentary lives. They sit all day at work, and when they come home, they turn on the TV and sit some more. Such people would naturally have very different imbalances. They might feel dull and lethargic, or have slow digestion, or put on weight—all symptoms associated with a fundamental Kapha imbalance. The personalized program that they would receive would be completely different from Bonnie's.

In Maharishi Ayur-Veda health care, there is no one program that suits everyone. Everyone's situation is different, and these differences help determine each person's unique needs. The Maharishi Ayur-Veda tradition offers practical knowledge to help create an ideal state of balanced health for everyone.

The chart on the following pages summarizes some of the characteristics of Vata, Pitta and Kapha.

91

Characteristics of Vata, Pitta and Kapha

Vata

When in balance:	When out of balance:
vibrant, lively	restless, unsettled
clear and alert mind	light, interrupted sleep
flexible, resilient	easily fatigued
imaginative, sensitive	constipated
cheerful, optimistic	anxious, worried
regular habits	underweight

What causes an imbalance in Vata:

irregular routine	excessive mental work
staying up late	traveling
cold, dry weather	accident or injury

Pitta

When in balance:	When out of balance:
warm, loving, contented	skin rashes, other skin diseases
enjoys meeting challenges	prematurely gray or thinning hair
strong digestion	irritable, angry and impatient
efficient in activity	demanding, critical, perfectionist
articulate and precise in speech	heartburn, ulcers, digestive problems
sharp intellect	finds hot weather unbearable

What causes an imbalance in Pitta:	
excessive heat or exposure to the sun time pressure, stressful deadlines	excessive activity, overwork skipping meals alcohol, smoking improper diet

Kapha

When in balance:	When out of balance:
strong, full of vitality affectionate, generous, kind, forgiving solid, powerful build natural resistance to disease good memory full of dignity and courage	complacent, dull, lethargic oily skin, allergies, congestion slow digestion, tendency to gain weight possessive, emotionally attached intolerant of the cold and damp inability to accept change

What causes an imbalance in Kapha:	
oversleeping overeating eating too many heavy, sweet or oily foods	insufficient exercise not enough variety in life cold, wet weather

Everything in Nature

Most people are fascinated by the knowledge of Vata, Pitta and Kapha, and can't wait to apply it more specifically to themselves. My patients often experience a real "ah-ha" when I explain how Vata, Pitta and Kapha work in their minds and bodies. They are always eager to know more. The knowledge makes sense; it intuitively fits their own understanding.

The knowledge of Vata, Pitta and Kapha is as old as the knowledge of life, as old as the laws of nature that govern life and living. And the beauty of this age-old system is that it is universally applicable. It describes everything in nature as well as ourselves. What's inside is also outside—there is only one continuum of life.

Vata, Pitta and Kapha govern the flow of nature's intelligence and help define the cycles and rhythms of nature. You will find them operating in each time of day, each season and each environment.

For example, Vata governs the early morning hours. If you wake up early (as recommended in this system of health care) you carry the light and lively qualities of Vata into the day with you, and your day will be more productive.

Pitta, being hot, governs the heat of the day. When you eat your main meal at noontime, you take advantage of the increased Pitta quality that predominates (both inside and outside) when the sun is highest in the sky, and your food will be digested that much more efficiently.

Kapha time is in the early evening, after the sun sets. It's the Kapha principle that makes it easier to fall asleep when you go to bed early, and makes your sleep deeper and more refreshing.

Vata is the principle most alive in the bitter dry cold of winter. Pitta governs the hot summertime. Kapha is associated with the heavy, cool, rainy days of spring. If you have a Vata or a Kapha imbalance, you tend to feel cold inside all the time, so the added coldness of winter and early spring may bother you. You may find yourself yearning for the warm sunny days of summer.

Our physical environment reflects the qualities of Vata, Pitta and Kapha, too. Vata is "airy." Pitta is "fiery" by nature. Kapha is associated with water and earth.

Vata can be found especially in high, dry, windy, rough or mountainous places. The desert, with its unrelenting heat and not a cloud in the sky, is intensely Pitta. Those who have a Pitta imbalance are usually miserable in hot desert climates and naturally gravitate toward environments that are more balancing for them. The oceanfront, with its cool, heavy, moist air and fogs blowing in from the sea, is very Kapha by nature.

Vata, Pitta and Kapha even apply to the foods we eat. Bitter greens, dry beans, and ice-cold drinks, for example, have mostly Vata qualities. When we eat them, they naturally increase the Vata principle in our minds and bodies. Hot, spicy food increases Pitta. Fried foods and rich desserts loaded with butter and sugar increase Kapha. When we know what foods have Vata, Pitta and Kapha qualities, then we can choose foods that provide more of what we need.

The qualities of Vata, Pitta and Kapha are found in people, in plants, in animals, in minerals—in everything around us. When we understand how Vata, Pitta and Kapha are "outside" as well as "inside," then it's easy to understand how we can use anything and everything in nature to help create inner balance. The Vata, Pitta and Kapha outside can be used to complement and enliven the Vata, Pitta and Kapha inside. The Maharishi Ayur-Veda system provides complete knowledge of how to use the gifts of nature wisely to help create ideal health.

Summary

Vata, Pitta and Kapha, the three main organizing principles of nature, govern all of nature, as well as the functioning of our minds and bodies. Maharishi Ayur-Veda health care provides complete knowledge of how Vata, Pitta and Kapha work together in each person, and how to create and maintain an ideal state of balance.

Chapter Fourteen

Pulse Diagnosis

At some point during your first Maharishi Ayur-Veda consultation, your doctor will ask to take your pulse. Placing the fingertips of his first three fingers precisely on your wrist, he will delicately but firmly press. He is not testing cardiovascular vitality; he is not counting beats per minute. Using the most sensitive instruments of all—his own fingertips and his informed judgment—he is gaining valuable information about the subtle workings of your mind and body.

For thousands of years, doctors trained in the art and science of pulse diagnosis have used this technique as a primary tool to learn more about their patients' needs. The beauty of pulse diagnosis is that it gives a comprehensive picture of a patient's state of balance and imbalance. The pulse can reveal important information—to one who is trained to feel it and understand what it conveys.

What exactly does your physician feel? He feels the different qualities of Vata, Pitta and Kapha as reflected in your pulse. The Vata pulse—like the Vata principle—is quick, light and changeable. The Pitta pulse is pulsing and energetic. The Kapha pulse glides along smoothly and quietly. He also evaluates the strength of Vata, Pitta and Kapha, and assesses the degree of balance at that particular time.

Everyone's pulse is different. And each person's pulse varies over time, reflecting factors that change and influence one during the day, in different seasons, and throughout a lifetime. For example, your pulse will have a different quality before and after a meal; it will feel different when you are twenty years, fifty years, eighty years. Your physician will feel these differences, and understand what they mean.

Moreover, he is trained to detect specific imbalances in Vata, Pitta and Kapha that are responsible for symptoms of disease. For example, he might feel a disturbance in the Vata pulse that indicates a profound Vata imbalance. This might explain why you can't fall asleep at night, no matter how you toss and turn. Or perhaps he feels a disturbance in your Pitta pulse, which indicates a Pitta imbalance. This would explain your problems with digestion, or why you have acne.

The advantage of this system of diagnosis is that it personalizes your symptoms to YOU. Your indigestion may be caused by a Vata imbalance; another person's indigestion may be caused by an imbalance in Pitta. A third person's indigestion may be caused by an imbalance in Kapha. The symptom is the same—indigestion—but the treatment will be different, depending on whether it is a Vata, Pitta or Kapha imbalance. Your physician will determine accurately through the pulse the root cause of your symptoms and prescribe a therapeutic program that addresses you and your unique needs.

A Boon to Prevention

Maharishi Ayur-Veda pulse diagnosis does not stop at identifying the root cause of your symptoms. Your physician is also trained to detect subtle imbalances in Vata, Pitta and Kapha—before they manifest into symptoms of disease. These imbalances are the result of subtle deviations in the expression of the body's inner intelligence.

Imbalances start quietly, almost imperceptibly. But left unchecked, they continue to grow, and inevitably cause problems on a gross level. The beauty of pulse diagnosis is that it reveals imbalances in their beginning stages, when they are still easy to catch and correct. It's easy to nip a problem in the bud; it's much harder—and takes longer—to correct an imbalance that has grown into a full-blown disease.

What a boon to preventive health care! What an elegant solution to the problem doctors have faced throughout the ages! Everyone agrees that the best chance we have to control disease lies in discovering it early, but until now there was no way to detect the beginning stages of disease. With Maharishi Ayur-Veda pulse diagnosis we now have such a way.

Moreover, once subtle imbalances are detected, the Maharishi Ayur-Veda system offers a complete range of therapies to correct them. Sometimes all it takes is extra rest, or eating more foods with a particular taste. Sometimes an herbal supplement is recommended, or a change in daily routine, or a combination of these therapies. But whatever the approach, it's easier when the imbalance has just begun.

More on Vata, Pitta, Kapha

When your physician takes your pulse on the most superficial level, he actually detects three distinct pulses, one under each of his first three fingers. But there is more to it than that. On a deeper and more subtle level of the pulse, he also detects the state of balance or imbalance of the various components of Vata, Pitta and Kapha. There are five components or subdivisions to each principle, which are associated with specific functions in the body. Knowledge gained from feeling the pulse on this level of detail is so precise that a doctor can identify what area of the body has accumulated an imbalance.

For example, one of the most important subdivisions of Vata is called *Apana Vata*. Apana Vata is located in the lower abdomen, and it governs the elimination of wastes and reproduction. When Apana Vata is balanced, the elimination of toxins is regular and complete, and reproductive functions are vital and problem-free. Moreover, a strong Apana Vata helps keep all of our energies more settled inside, so that our breath is softer, our minds clearer, our thoughts more purposeful, and our activity more productive.

An imbalance in Apana Vata can be at the root of many different complaints. Some are obviously associated with the lower abdomen, such as urinary tract infections and menstrual disorders. But some are not so obvious. A long-term imbalance in Apana Vata can sometimes upset even Pitta or Kapha. The symptoms would then seem more like Pitta or Kapha imbalances, but Maharishi Ayur-Veda pulse diagnosis would reveal the true source of the problem in Vata.

Through the pulse, your doctor can evaluate the functioning of Vata, Pitta, Kapha and their various subdivisions. And other aspects of the pulse help give your doctor additional information. For example, your doctor can assess your overall vitality, the strength of your digestion, and the functioning of various tissues in your body. All of this information is valuable and helps him understand what you need.

It takes only a few seconds and a simple touch on the wrist, but it is your physician's most valuable diagnostic tool.

The Touch That Helps Heal

We have mentioned the saying, "The whole is more than the sum of its parts." With Maharishi Ayur-Veda pulse diagnosis, another principle is at work—"The whole is contained in every part." The whole of the mind and body is contained in the subtle variations of the pulse. Through the traditional knowledge of Maharishi Ayur-Veda health care we know what each variation means. It's as if the body were speaking a kind of secret language. The Maharishi Ayur-Veda tradition provides the key that unlocks the code.

Is knowledge of the pulse esoteric? Only as esoteric as a science tested by thousands of years of experience. Like everything in this system of health care, it works. It has passed the test of time and proven its worth.

Doctors trained in Maharishi Ayur-Veda health care (when compared to other physicians) generally seem to depend less on routine medical testing procedures—which are often expensive, prolonged, invasive and painful. They tend to rely more on the information they receive through the pulse and their patients' personal histories and experiences. As needed, they complement this information with modern technological investigations.

Routine lab results cannot provide the same information as the pulse. Modern technology, as sophisticated as it is, is not refined enough to detect subtle imbalances. Conventional tests, however, are used to corroborate information obtained through pulse diagnosis and can be additional tools in the management and follow-up of complicated disease. Modern technology complements the Maharishi Ayur-Veda approach by providing specific investigations to obtain specific results.

It is said that part of the cure is in the healing touch of the physician as he takes your pulse. Maharishi Ayur-Veda pulse diagnosis, in and of itself, can be therapeutic. Why is this so? Because taking the pulse is a quiet process. In taking the pulse, the doctor takes recourse to his own settled level of awareness. Pulse diagnosis is enlivening to consciousness—both the consciousness of the doctor and the consciousness of the patient. And—as we have seen with every Maharishi Ayur-Veda therapy—it is enlivened consciousness that naturally, spontaneously, effortlessly corrects imbalances from within and brings wholeness and perfection to life.

Self-Pulse Reading

If the touch of a properly trained physician can be therapeutic, imagine how much more enlivening your own sense of touch can be—if properly trained. And in fact, courses in self-pulse reading are offered through Maharishi Ayur-Veda Universities and Schools.[1] These courses teach you how to take your own pulse, how to interpret what you feel, and how to adjust your preventive daily routine to help maintain an ideal state of balance.

The advantage of taking your own pulse is that you can monitor your health on a daily basis. You have the diagnostic tool, and you have the knowledge you need to take care of yourself and your changing needs. Moreover, taking the pulse is like an advanced technique for the development of consciousness, in that it allows your awareness to settle down to a very refined state of quiet alertness. Self-pulse reading nourishes the inner self, completes the circle of self-knowledge, and brings greater self-sufficiency to health care.

---

[1] See chapter nineteen for a list of Maharishi Ayur-Veda Universities and Schools.

Summary

The pulse is like a window giving a comprehensive view of your mind and body. Through Maharishi Ayur-Veda pulse diagnosis, physicians can determine the degree of balance or imbalance in Vata, Pitta and Kapha, identify the root cause of existing symptoms, and identify subtle imbalances that might cause problems in the future. The knowledge of the pulse has broad implications for the diagnosis, treatment and prevention of disease.

Chapter Fifteen

What to Expect

L et me preface this chapter by mentioning what NOT to expect. Do not expect assembly-line medicine. Do not expect to wait for hours in a doctor's office only to get a few minutes of the doctor's time and a handful of prescriptions.

Expect to have enough time to discuss your situation. Expect to be listened to. Expect to learn a lot about yourself and why you feel the way you do.

Expect to have questions. And expect them to be answered. Gaining more knowledge and intellectual understanding is considered very important and necessary to the healing process in the Maharishi Ayur-Veda approach.

In the Maharishi Ayur-Veda system, you are an equal partner with your physician in correcting imbalances and creating ideal health. Your doctor will depend on you to provide valuable information about yourself and your symptoms of disease. He or she will take the time to diagnose you properly and provide a personalized program of treatment. Your doctor will expect you, in turn, to follow your new program over time and provide important feedback on your experiences.

Your First Visit

Your relationship with your new physician usually starts with an initial evaluation. In this first visit, your doctor gets to know you, so you may be asked to fill out a medical history form and a questionnaire asking basic questions about yourself. This background information helps orient the doctor to YOU and your unique situation.

Central to your first visit is the doctor's pulse diagnosis. Using this time-honored and effective technique, the doctor will determine the degree of balance and imbalance in Vata, Pitta and Kapha, which will help to disclose the root cause of your symptoms of disease. With this knowledge, he or she can then begin to prescribe therapies to correct the problem.

In Maharishi Ayur-Veda health care, there is no one solution. There are many! Whatever the problem, it is addressed from every possible angle—through the mind, the body, the intellect, the emotions, behavior and the environment. All Maharishi Ayur-Veda treatments work together to create the greatest possible therapeutic effect.

The Maharishi Ayur-Veda health program is not just herbal supplements. Your recommendations will include herbal formulas, but there will always be other approaches. All of the treatments are natural and take the whole system into account. No one area benefits at the expense of any other.

Expect to feel nourished and strengthened as your underlying problems are gently, naturally corrected. Expect to notice side benefits rather than side effects.

Expect to have fun with your new program. Maharishi Ayur-Veda health care is all about enjoying more fullness in life, so nothing in your treatment should cause strain or discomfort. It may take some attention, and it may take a commitment of time, but the rewards are worth it.

This approach essentially calls for some change in lifestyle, but it does not have to be sudden or painful. The transition can be gradual and comfortable. You can proceed at your own pace, starting with suggestions that are easy to incorporate into your existing routine, and add new recommendations as you feel better and your life improves.

Both Prevention and Treatment

The purpose of a Maharishi Ayur-Veda consultation is two-fold. The first is prevention of disease. According to this tradition of health care, disease does not develop overnight, and it is the primary goal of this approach to prevent disease from happening in the first place and to nip any potential problem in the bud. Treatment of disease becomes necessary only when appropriate preventive measures have not been taken.

The second purpose of a consultation is to take corrective action if disease has already manifested. But even as it provides treatment, Maharishi Ayur-Veda health care will always emphasize prevention of further disease. As it corrects the problem it will strengthen the system to avoid future imbalances.

Although the experience of disease may bring you to the doorstep of the Maharishi Ayur-Veda approach, it is the knowledge of how you can create and maintain health that will keep you interested for life. As you follow your doctor's advice and begin to choose better foods, live a more natural lifestyle, and benefit from many other Maharishi Ayur-Veda therapies, you will grow in the realization that the key to perfect health lies in your very own hands. The traditional knowledge will give you control over your health that you never dreamed was possible.

In my practice, I usually see patients for an initial consultation, and then follow-up visits as needed. Within a few weeks, patients are well on their way to better health, and self-sufficient in the knowledge of how to prevent further imbalances. Still, I encourage them to return for preventive check-ups every three months. Regular follow-ups ensure steady progress on the path to perfect health.

The Maharishi Ayur-Veda system of health care offers all the knowledge you need to create and maintain an ideal state of health. Your doctor will provide basic and essential information, and courses in this knowledge are offered through Maharishi Vedic Universities and Maharishi Ayur-Veda Universities. For more information on these courses, see chapter nineteen.

In a nutshell, what can you expect? Expect your health to improve. Expect to start enjoying life more. Expect that life will change—in subtle ways, in surprising ways, in dramatic ways. The Maharishi Ayur-Veda approach is not a magic bullet; it is not an instant cure. But in the long run, you may find—like many others before you—that the magic it offers can truly transform your life.

Summary

With the Maharishi Ayur-Veda system of health care you can expect to work hand in hand with your doctor to create perfect health. While this tradition offers treatment for disease, its primary focus is prevention and giving you the necessary knowledge to take control of your own health.

Part IV

A Vision of Possibilities

In Part III we discussed the specialized knowledge that a physician trained in Maharishi Ayur-Veda health care can provide. Using Maharishi Ayur-Veda pulse diagnosis and other diagnostic procedures, your doctor will determine exactly what you need to restore balance in Vata, Pitta and Kapha. When the system is balanced, then symptoms of disease automatically disappear.

All Maharishi Ayur-Veda treatments are tailored to each person's needs. Because they address fundamental imbalances that are unique to you and your situation, they can succeed in providing real and lasting benefits.

In Part IV, we present a vision of possibilities with the Maharishi Ayur-Veda approach. In chapter sixteen we tell the stories of actual patients who have used Maharishi Ayur-Veda health care. Chapter seventeen presents the questions most frequently asked, and their answers.

In chapter eighteen, we discuss scientific research on Maharishi Ayur-Veda health care. Maharishi Mahesh Yogi has said, "Through the window of science we see the dawn of the Age of Enlightenment." It is largely due to the substantial body of scientific research done on the Transcendental Meditation technique and other Maharishi Ayur-Veda approaches that we envision a fundamental change in the trends of time promising a better quality of life for all. Chapter eighteen presents a sampling of the research that has been conducted over the past twenty-five years, and draws some initial conclusions about its long-term and far-reaching implications.

Finally, in chapter nineteen, we will tell you how to find out more about this age-old system of health care.

Chapter Sixteen

Maharishi Ayur-Veda
Health Care Helped Me

There is a saying that the teacher always learns more than the student. Similarly, as a physician practicing Maharishi Ayur-Veda health care, I feel that the doctor always gains more than the patient.

Through my Maharishi Ayur-Veda practice, I have grown personally to understand health and disease from a new perspective. I have learned to see and treat the patient as a whole person. And I feel that this holistic approach is the need of our time. Through this system of health care, we have the chance to create health and happiness—and gain knowledge of life itself.

In my practice, I always feel that I am growing along with my patients. Together, our awareness evolves to new levels.

The purpose of this chapter, which summarizes the experiences of a few of my patients, is not to make claims of superiority over other systems of medicine. It is my personal experience that the integrated approach of Maharishi Ayur-Veda health care with conventional medicine is highly useful for both physician and patient. And I fully support Maharishi Mahesh Yogi in his initiative to launch Maharishi Colleges of Vedic Medicine throughout the world. This is the wave of the future that will bring new hope to all.

Forever Healthy as the title for this book reflects the hope I feel for my patients. I chose this title because I felt it was appropriate and truthful to the Maharishi Ayur-Veda tradition. Some people may find the idea fanciful or unrealistic. But as I review the age-old texts of Ayur-Veda I realize again that the idea of being healthy and vital forever is a real possibility, especially when the Maharishi Ayur-Veda system of health care is introduced before conception and is applied throughout one's entire life. Knowing that there is this real possibility, I feel responsible to share it with you. And I invite you, in turn, to consider this possibility for yourself, and to take heart in the knowledge that others have enjoyed perfect health before you.

When patients first came to me, they came because they were not happy with the care they had been receiving. Later, many patients came because they desired the natural and holistic therapies of the Maharishi Ayur-Veda tradition. These patients, usually well-educated and well-informed, simply wanted something better—an approach in harmony with nature. Now I also see many patients who come because they have been referred by other patients. When someone they know gets better, they naturally want to try that approach too, even though they know nothing about it before their first appointment.

But no matter why they come, my patients all want one thing— that is, good health. Their focus is on health, not just on disease. And as a physician practicing Maharishi Ayur-Veda health care, I have learned that the focus should always be on health—even though the way to create health is to treat the underlying imbalances that cause disease.

No single physician or medical system can guarantee everyone cures for all disease. As you know, disease is a complex process and develops over time. The treatment outcome varies with the stage and severity of the disease, the course of the treatment and the compliance of the patient.

However, that said, in my experience practicing Maharishi Ayur-Veda health care, patients begin to enjoy a more holistic value of health on a very personal level. Changes in diet and daily routine, herbal formulas, practice of the Transcendental Meditation technique, rejuvenation therapies, etc.—all their Maharishi Ayur-Veda treatments create subtle and profound changes that result in a deep inner experience of improved health, more happiness, greater peace and a sense of inner balance.

I have also found that this personal experience of health grows over time. In the beginning it may be simply an abatement of symptoms. But with time and growth in understanding, true health begins to be experienced on all levels—body, mind and spirit.

Here are the summaries of real case histories from my own experience practicing Maharishi Ayur-Veda health care. They are included in this book as concrete examples of how one can benefit from this approach, and also to give you a vision of possibilities.

Steven

Steven White[1] suffered from severe allergic reactions. For as long as he could remember, his allergies would begin in August and last until the first frost. During allergy season, he experienced itchy eyes and nasal irritation, and was treated frequently for sinus infections and strep throat. His symptoms included severe headaches and gastrointestinal cramps, with episodes of diarrhea. He was often tired and slept for long periods of time. He was also overweight and wanted to lose more than 60 pounds.

Steven had tried most conventional therapies, including desensitization shots for many years. He felt that his drowsiness and lack of energy were probably caused by prescription medicines. In his search for relief, Steven tried many alternate therapies, but the results were inadequate.

After his Maharishi Ayur-Veda consultation Steven began the practice of the Transcendental Meditation technique. Immediately he reported that during meditation his symptoms lessened. He also started taking Maharishi Ayur-Veda herbal formulas and adjusted his daily routine and diet in accord with my recommendations. Over the next few weeks Steven reported that his symptoms associated with seasonal allergies were minimal to none.

After a few months Steven stopped taking the herbal formulas, but he continued with his Maharishi Ayur-Veda daily routine and diet.

---

[1] To respect patient confidentiality, actual names have been changed in the case histories selected for this chapter.

He found that seasonal adjustments to his diet were particularly helpful in eliminating weight gain. As of the writing of this book, Steven is still very regular with his Maharishi Ayur-Veda routine, and has maintained a 60-pound weight loss. He has been free of all symptoms of disease—including seasonal allergies—for over three years.

Alex

Fourteen-year old Alex Kern was brought to my office by his parents, who were desperate to help their child recover from asthma and depression.

When I spoke with Alex, he told me that severe asthma symptoms began just after his tenth birthday. He complained about taking daily medication to relieve his symptoms. He was despondent, and showed no signs of the usual teenage vigor.

Alex first started taking Maharishi Ayur-Veda herbal formulas to help balance his physiology. Then, with little enthusiasm and no expectations, he learned and began practicing the Transcendental Meditation technique.

When I saw him a month later, Alex showed more energy and enthusiasm. He said that he enjoyed his twice-daily practice of meditation. His parents reported that Alex was breathing more easily and using substantially less asthma medication. At this visit, I added additional therapies to his Maharishi Ayur-Veda routine.

Three months later, Alex required conventional asthma medication to help him breathe only on rare occasions. His breathless asthmatic episodes had subsided considerably. He had a youthful joy and vigor about him and there were no indications of depression.

Nearly three years later, Alex has remained stable and is looking forward to attending a good college.

Janet

Janet Smith's menstrual periods had become a monthly torture of severe cramping, debilitating headaches, and an extremely heavy flow. Nothing she had tried to alleviate her symptoms had ever given her total relief.

The owner of a natural foods store in upstate New York, Janet decided to try the Maharishi Ayur-Veda approach at the recommendation of a customer who had controlled his high blood pressure with the help of Maharishi Ayur-Veda therapies.

When she came to see me, I prescribed a complete Maharishi Ayur-Veda program, including the practice of the Transcendental Meditation technique, special exercises, herbal supplements, and dietary changes such as the elimination of caffeine and hot, spicy foods.

After two months on her new program, Janet reported that her menstrual discomfort had abated significantly.

After two and a half years, Janet still sees me for seasonal check-ups, and feels that her overall health has improved greatly with the Maharishi Ayur-Veda approach.

Barbara

At age fifteen, Barbara Broyd was a nervous and worried teenager who complained of painful stomach disorders. The pain in her stomach had bothered her for the last five years. Before she came to see me, appropriate medical testing had been done, but it showed no obvious pathology.

I immediately prescribed a diet, herbal formulas and other Maharishi Ayur-Veda therapies to help correct Barbara's underlying imbalances.

One week after she came to me for her initial consultation, Barbara learned the practice of the Transcendental Meditation technique. Very soon after that, she reported feeling more secure inside and less troubled by her stomach complaints. Over the next several weeks, her symptoms began to subside in a dramatic way.

A few months after her first visit, Barbara visited a Maharishi Ayur-Veda Medical Center for seasonal rejuvenation treatment. After her treatment, she reported that her stomach ailments abated.

She also experienced improvement in other areas—fewer headaches, for example.

She also said that she enjoyed more energy and stamina, and that her symptoms of anxiety and worry were substantially reduced. As her practice of meditation continued over time, Barbara reported that all experience of discomfort and disease eventually disappeared.

Thomas

Thomas Gill sought my advice at age 41 because of severe and chronic pain. He told me that since the time he was 20 he had experienced excruciating pain in his wrists, knees and shoulders. He had been diagnosed with chronic rheumatoid arthritis and was in pain most of every day. Many times a month Thomas was in so much pain that he could not get out of bed.

He had used all forms of available medical treatment to alleviate his suffering, and had even undergone back surgery some years earlier. Thomas had also tried alternative remedies, but none freed him from the constant experience of pain.

I immediately gave Thomas personalized diet instructions, and prescribed a complete Maharishi Ayur-Veda program, including herbal supplements and the regular practice of the Transcendental Meditation technique.

Within a few weeks the swelling in his joints was greatly reduced and he was experiencing greater mobility. He was able to walk around and perform minimal work. In a month he even felt well enough to travel out of the country. He still experienced some pain in his larger joints, but he was no longer disabled.

Thomas continues his regular practice of the TM technique, and also does special Maharishi Ayur-Veda exercises to improve his mobility.

Gregory

At age ten, Gregory Brandon weighed more than 130 pounds—

approximately 50 pounds too much for his age and build. His parents had taken him to various pediatricians and specialists over the years without much success. Gregory's pediatrician referred him to me because he knew they wanted more help for their child.

Gregory had received complete testing for metabolic and endocrine disorders, and the lab results were normal. When I saw him, Gregory was taking prescription medicine but was still gaining weight at the rate of two pounds per week. He was experiencing fatigue and could no longer participate in sports. He also had associated sinus problems and headaches. Moreover, the thought of additional tests and investigative procedures made Gregory afraid.

I immediately recommended a daily routine and diet to help restore balance, and prescribed Maharishi Ayur-Veda herbal formulas and special exercises. I also recommended that he start the practice of the TM technique. I advised his parents not to weigh him for a while, and told Gregory not to worry about his weight and to enjoy himself.

Upon his next visit a month later, his parents reported that Gregory's sinus problems had cleared up completely, that he was showing increased vigor and energy, and that he was taking a renewed interest in sports. They even volunteered that his study habits had improved.

During the first month, Gregory stopped putting on additional weight. During the second month, he lost three pounds as he grew one-half inch taller. By the third month, Gregory had lost five pounds. After six months he had grown two inches taller and his weight had remained stable.

Two years later Gregory continues to see me for regular check-ups. He loves football and is playing on his school's football team. He meditates regularly and continues his simple daily exercises. Although he has a big frame and will always be large, there is no gross imbalance. Both Gregory and his parents report their pleasure at the results of the Maharishi Ayur-Veda treatment.

Andrew

Andrew Fells came to me at age 37. He had experienced 17 years of conventional drug therapy for manic depressive illness (bipolar depression). At the time of his first Maharishi Ayur-Veda consultation he was also being treated for alcohol abuse.

Moreover, Andrew had a history of frequent urinary and kidney problems which he attributed to side effects from his current treatment.

Andrew first learned the practice of the Transcendental Meditation technique and, inspired by his experiences, decided to try other Maharishi Ayur-Veda therapies as well. After two months of following a complete Maharishi Ayur-Veda program, Andrew reported increased enjoyment and stability in life, and his need for conventional medicine was sharply reduced. His chronic kidney pain and other secondary symptoms had subsided. He even commented on his improved quality of sleep. Working closely with his primary care physician, I was able to reduce much of Andrew's prescription medication, and eventually he needed only one.

Within four months Andrew's life had completely turned around. His abuse of alcohol had ceased, he had started a new job, and in his free time he began writing a novel.

Two and a half years later Andrew is still doing well with the integrated approach of Maharishi Ayur-Veda health care and conventional medicine.

Alice

Alice Burns, age 53, sought my advice to alleviate symptoms associated with her thyroid condition. She was especially concerned about her weight gain.

I recommended daily practice of the Transcendental Meditation technique, a daily routine that included gentle exercise, and Maharishi Ayur-Veda herbal formulas in addition to her conventional treatment. After a few weeks she reported that many of her symptoms of discomfort were eliminated, that she was experiencing more energy, and that she had begun to lose weight gradually (and, as it turned out, permanently).

Alice continued to monitor her thyroid functioning regularly with conventional lab testing. In two months, her thyroid began to shrink. At the end of three months her conventional thyroid medicine was reduced by 50%.

Doreen

Doreen Verns had been diagnosed with ulcerative colitis at an early age. After learning the practice of the Transcendental Meditation technique at age 43, she experienced a two-year remission in her symptoms.

Then she became irregular in her meditation practice and her symptoms gradually returned. She experienced reduced appetite, weight loss, cramps and debilitating diarrhea with the passing of blood. Doreen finally sought Maharishi Ayur-Veda treatment to eliminate the root cause of her illness.

At my advice, Doreen began meditating regularly again. I also prescribed changes in diet and the addition of specific Maharishi Ayur-Veda herbal formulas. Within one month she reported feeling much improved and her conventional medicine was reduced. After four months she was once again in remission. She reported experiencing increased energy and good health.

After three years, Doreen is still symptom-free and comes to me only for regular preventive check-ups.

John

John Light was diagnosed with lymphocytic leukemia at age 53. After his diagnosis John underwent chemotherapy, which left him so exhausted that he feared he would never fully recover from the treatment. He decided at that time to seek alternate therapies.

John had practiced the Transcendental Meditation technique for many years and was interested in working in harmony with his body's

119

own inner intelligence. He came to me for the Maharishi Ayur-Veda approach.

John received a personalized Maharishi Ayur-Veda program and, at my advice, went for seasonal rejuvenation treatments. Now John enjoys an active life once again. One of his favorite activities is hiking and mountain climbing. He reports that he has never felt better in his life—including before his illness was diagnosed.

After five years, John continues his practice of Transcendental Meditation and goes for seasonal rejuvenation treatments regularly. His white blood cell count is still slightly elevated, but he has no other symptoms of disease and takes no medication. John still regularly sees his oncologist, who is very supportive of John's involvement with Maharishi Ayur-Veda health care and keeps me posted with John's progress reports.

Liz

Dr. Liz Brown, director of a child education program at a prominent university, experienced preliminary symptoms of multiple sclerosis off and on for more than 15 years. Then she came down with optic neuritis and faced the real possibility that her symptoms would develop into full-fledged disease. It was then that she decided to try the Maharishi Ayur-Veda approach. She followed a complete Maharishi Ayur-Veda program and went for seasonal rejuvenation treatments regularly.

Using various Maharishi Ayur-Veda therapies, Dr. Brown has managed to stay well enough to continue with her demanding work. She says, "I feel that the Ayurvedic treatment modalities I've undertaken have allowed me to be extremely healthy within the limitations posed by a disease that leaves most people incapable of working. . . . I haven't had to be hospitalized or, as is most often the case, to take steroids to avert some of the more severe complications of multiple sclerosis. I feel that I've experienced a definite decrease in the morbidity of the disease."

120

Jim

Jim Carpenter, a writer and lecturer living in the Midwest, had various health complaints, including heart palpitations and a cough that just wouldn't go away. Jim consulted a cardiologist and a pulmonary specialist, but neither were able to provide relief.

Jim felt that his whole system was flashing red lights. It was one disease after another—a cold, then flu, then digestive problems—and in general he had no energy.

In addition, Jim watched helplessly as his cholesterol level climbed 14 points over a nine-month period, in spite of the fact that he was carefully maintaining a strict, low-fat diet.

Jim tried Maharishi Ayur-Veda health care as a last resort, and started with a week-long seasonal rejuvenation treatment at a regional Maharishi Ayur-Veda Medical Center. After just one week, his cough and heart palpitations disappeared completely and his blood cholesterol level dropped 54 points. With the help of a Maharishi Ayur-Veda home preventive program, Jim has remained in good health ever since.

Final Comments

In my experience, Jim Carpenter's case is all too common. A patient has symptoms, and he doesn't know why. His doctor tries to provide an answer, but often it is unsatisfactory. The patient turns to Maharishi Ayur-Veda health care as a last resort.

Jim's story is particularly dramatic in that just one week of treatment was enough to turn the tide. Jim himself expressed delight that all of his symptoms disappeared in one stroke—and also astonishment that no attention was given to his symptoms per se. This is because the Maharishi Ayur-Veda approach focuses on eliminating the root cause of symptoms—underlying imbalances. It is far more effective to deal with a problem at its root. Even when symptoms seem very different and unrelated on the surface, they are often caused by one fundamental imbalance. When the imbalance is corrected, symptoms disappear on their own.

It is also common for patients to tell me that, although they don't have consistent symptoms or a disease they can identify, still they don't feel quite right. Their energy level is low, or they get tired, or they feel a lot of anxiety. Often there is a series of small complaints—aches and pains, headaches, a flu that seems to linger. This kind of complaint is often dismissed by conventional doctors as a kind of neurosis or hypochondria. But physicians trained in Maharishi Ayur-Veda health care take all such experiences very seriously. Often a patient senses the development of an imbalance long before disease becomes evident on a gross level. Such subtle imbalances can be verified easily using Maharishi Ayur-Veda pulse diagnosis, and corrected using Maharishi Ayur-Veda therapies.

In my experience, most patients benefit in some way from the Maharishi Ayur-Veda approach. In addition (as was noted in several case histories), this approach works very successfully with conventional medicine in the treatment of many chronic diseases.

Moreover, patients who have been treated successfully with conventional medicine, but who still experience some discomfort, and patients who experience side effects from their treatment often benefit from using Maharishi Ayur-Veda health care. In such cases, a patient usually continues with conventional medication and treatment while adding Maharishi Ayur-Veda therapies. Over time, he often requires less medication, and in some cases is able to discontinue conventional treatment altogether.

It is important to understand that each case is individual, and that with serious and chronic diseases, time is necessary. For example, a patient who has suffered from chronic asthma for fifteen to twenty years may need several weeks of Maharishi Ayur-Veda treatment before he experiences any relief, and several months of treatment before he can consider reducing his conventional medication. But patients who commit to the Maharishi Ayur-Veda approach will start to regain balance and enjoy a growing experience of inner health from the very first day.

Your physician has your comfort and safety in mind, and will plan a Maharishi Ayur-Veda program that will ensure steady, sure progress on the path to perfect health.

Summary

In my practice, most patients respond to Maharishi Ayur-Veda treatment, either alone or in conjunction with conventional medicine. The time necessary to produce an effect is highly individual, depending on the patient and the nature of the disease. But the experience of my patients indicates that positive results can be expected.

Chapter Seventeen

Questions and Answers

Q. What is Maharishi Ayur-Veda health care?

A. *Ayur-Veda* literally means "knowledge of life." *Maharishi* literally means "great seer" or "enlightened sage." Maharishi Ayur-Veda health care is the age-old wisdom of life that has come down from the great seers of the ancient Vedic tradition. Specifically, it is complete knowledge about how to live a long, healthy and happy life.

In this generation, the traditional knowledge has been restored to its full value by Maharishi Mahesh Yogi, the founder of the Transcendental Meditation program. Now complete and true to its Vedic origins, Maharishi Ayur-Veda health care offers knowledge to bring fulfillment to all areas of life.

Q. What is the difference between Ayur-Veda and Maharishi Ayur-Veda health care?

A. Maharishi Ayur-Veda health care is complete Ayur-Veda. It emphasizes the vital role that development of consciousness plays in creating perfect health and bringing complete balance to life. All of the approaches of Maharishi Ayur-Veda health care give primary importance to the development of consciousness; all derive their effectiveness from enlivening pure consciousness and the body's inner intelligence.

Q. I am overwhelmed by all the different approaches of the Maharishi Ayur-Veda system. Where do I start? Will I benefit by using only one or two approaches?

A. You will certainly benefit by using just a part of the Maharishi Ayur-Veda system of health care. Discuss with your physician the most important approaches for you and start with one or two. All of the approaches work individually; they also work in conjunction with each other. The more approaches you use, the greater the overall effect.

The important thing is to start. People usually discover that trying even one approach makes it easier to incorporate others. Most of the therapies can be adapted easily to your current schedule and life-style. Moreover, you will find that the different therapies are highly enjoyable, and the benefits accumulate with time—so why wait?

Q. Do I have to practice the Transcendental Meditation technique in order to derive benefits from the Maharishi Ayur-Veda approach?

A. No. You do not have to practice the Transcendental Meditation technique to receive benefits from Maharishi Ayur-Veda health care. All of the approaches work independently, and you will receive benefits from any one of them. The practice of the TM technique is highly recommended, however, because it is the most powerful and holistic therapy of the Maharishi Ayur-Veda system. It improves your health as a whole because it gives the direct experience of pure consciousness, which nourishes and gives life to your mind and body.

Q. What makes the Transcendental Meditation technique different from other kinds of meditation?

A. The Transcendental Meditation technique is unique. All other kinds of meditation, while they may have some value, involve either concentration or contemplation, which keeps the mind active on the surface level of thought. They usually require some kind of mental effort or "trying."

The Transcendental Meditation technique requires no effort. It allows the conscious mind to settle down and experience its source— pure consciousness, or pure creative intelligence. The technique is easy to learn and enjoyable to practice, and produces a wide range of benefits. These benefits have been verified by extensive scientific research.

126

Dozens of scientific studies have compared the TM technique to other forms of meditation, relaxation techniques, and hypnosis. The studies found that it is far more effective at reducing anxiety, increasing self-actualization and improving both psychological and physical health.[1]

Q. How soon can I expect results from using the Maharishi Ayur-Veda approach?

A. All Maharishi Ayur-Veda therapies begin to produce results right away. From the moment you start, they begin to bring balance to the entire mind-body system. The time it takes to completely balance the mind and body and for you to notice the effects will vary with each individual. A lot depends on the nature of the individual and the nature and duration of the imbalance that needs to be corrected.

Q. I lead a very busy life. Does Maharishi Ayur-Veda health care take up a lot of time?

A. Maharishi Ayur-Veda health care does not have to take up a lot of time. It does take attention to fit various approaches into a busy schedule. But most people find that the attention they give to it is well rewarded by the increased energy, vitality, enjoyment and well-being that they feel throughout the day. And most people find that their Maharishi Ayur-Veda routine actually saves them time in the long run because they are more efficient in their activity and miss less work due to illness.

Your Maharishi Ayur-Veda routine should never be a strain. It is not the purpose of this tradition to add stress and strain to an already busy life! Often it is simply a matter of setting priorities. When you incorporate Maharishi Ayur-Veda approaches into your daily life, you will find that it's easier to set priorities and give attention to what's really important.

---

[1] For more information on scientific research see chapter eighteen.

Q. Is Maharishi Ayur-Veda health care something I need to do for the rest of my life, or can I use it just when I need it?

A. Health is your most valuable possession. You live with your state of health day in and day out. If anything is worth an investment of your time and attention, certainly your health is!

The Maharishi Ayur Veda tradition provides complete knowledge to help you maintain health and prevent disease. Once you know how to stay healthy using this approach, it becomes simply a matter of routine maintenance. Treatment modalities are always available if you need them.

Most of my patients find that they enjoy using the various Maharishi Ayur-Veda approaches, and that it's easy to continue with a preventive routine even after all their symptoms of disease have disappeared.

Q. Can I continue to take my prescription drugs while I use Maharishi Ayur-Veda therapies? Is there any conflict between conventional medicine and Maharishi Ayur-Veda health care?

A. You may certainly continue with your prescribed medications while you use Maharishi Ayur-Veda therapies; in fact, in most cases, this is the wise and safe thing to do. However, over time, you may find that you need less and less medication. Eventually you may be able to eliminate it altogether. It is important to follow the advice of your doctors when cutting back on the use of prescription drugs.

There is no conflict between Maharishi Ayur-Veda health care and conventional medicine. Doctors who are not trained in the Maharishi Ayur-Veda approach may not understand how well they can work together, but this is my daily experience. Please refer to chapter six and chapter sixteen for more information.

Q. Can Maharishi Ayur-Veda health care cure my high blood pressure (back pain, headaches, or any other ailment)?

A. In my experience, most patients can expect positive results from Maharishi Ayur-Veda treatment. The time it takes to provide relief will depend on the patient and the nature and duration of the disease. In situations where a disease is too advanced, and the time too little to effect a complete cure, even then my patients are always appreciative and grateful for the improved quality of life and clarity of consciousness that they experience with Maharishi Ayur-Veda health care.

Q. Can the Maharishi Ayur-Veda approach help with mental concerns such as anxiety, depression and fear?

A. According to the Maharishi Ayur-Veda tradition, mental concerns are just another set of symptoms indicating an underlying imbalance in the mind and body. When the imbalance is corrected, mental concerns often disappear just like other symptoms of disease.

In the Maharishi Ayur-Veda system, it is possible to treat mental problems with physical as well as mental approaches. This is because the mind and body are intimately connected. For example, it is very common for people with a fundamental Vata imbalance to have a lot of worries. After recommending that they learn the Transcendental Meditation technique, I often suggest simple changes in diet, so that their foods include more Vata-balancing tastes.

In the Maharishi Ayur-Veda tradition, it is not important to analyze the "reason" for worries. The reason, according to this tradition, is always the underlying imbalance, and once that is corrected, the worries disappear. The situation in life may not change, but the person's ability to handle that situation does change—for the better!

Q. Is Maharishi Ayur-Veda health care safe and effective for everyone? Can children use it? How about pregnant women?

A. Maharishi Ayur-Veda health care is recommended for everyone. No matter what your age or state of health, no matter where you live or what you believe, it offers safe and effective health care for your needs.

129

And the earlier you start, the better! Maharishi Ayur-Veda knowledge applies from the moment of conception. In fact, one of the most precious aspects of this tradition is the knowledge of how to make pregnancy and childbirth a comfortable and healthy experience for both mother and child. As always, and especially during pregnancy, it is important to work closely with your doctor and follow his or her recommendations.

In addition, there are herbal formulas designed just for children's special needs, and children as young as four can learn the children's Transcendental Meditation technique. My own experience is that children "take" to Maharishi Ayur-Veda knowledge very easily— sometimes more easily than their parents, who have many years of bad habits to undo! Children naturally understand basic principles of life when they are explained (such as getting enough rest to better enjoy their activity), and can be active participants in eating properly and following a good daily routine.

Q. How can I find out more about Maharishi Ayur-Veda health care? Where do I go from here?

A. Read on! The last chapter in this book will tell you how to find your nearest Maharishi Ayur-Veda University, your nearest doctor trained in Maharishi Ayur-Veda health care and your nearest teacher of the Transcendental Meditation technique. In addition, we have supplied information on other aspects of the Maharishi Vedic Approach to Health for those who are interested.

I encourage you to go on for more—and to apply this knowledge to your life. Learning new knowledge is valuable in and of itself, but the knowledge of Maharishi Ayur-Veda health care is meant to make a real difference in your day-to-day life.

I wish this book could give you everything you need, but the truth is, it can't. No book can assess your unique needs and give you a personalized program for better health. But it can give you a taste of what's available, describe the benefits that await you, and show you where to go for more. It is my hope that this book is a step for you in the right direction—towards better health and greater fulfillment in life.

130

Summary

In this chapter we presented the most frequently asked questions about Maharishi Ayur-Veda health care and their answers. For more information, see chapter nineteen.

Chapter Eighteen

Scientific Research:
Profound Benefits for Health

Heaven on Earth on the individual level will be characterized by perfect health, long life in bliss, and the ability to fulfill one's desires. Heaven on Earth on the collective level will be characterized by an indomitable influence of positivity, harmony, and peace in the family, community, nation, and the world. —Maharishi Mahesh Yogi

From the very beginning, Maharishi encouraged research on the Transcendental Meditation technique and other aspects of the Maharishi Ayur-Veda system, recognizing the importance of scientific research in validating this approach for a scientific age.

As long ago as 1964, Maharishi discussed the profound physiological changes that take place during the practice of the Transcendental Meditation technique. "About immortality on the physical level . . ." he said, "when the mind experiences finer realms of thought during meditation, then the metabolism is reduced. As the metabolism is reduced, the activity of the mind becomes finer and finer, and the metabolism becomes further reduced. The mind transcends and gets to that state of transcendental consciousness. Simultaneously the body, the mind, the entire functioning of the inner machinery, the whole metabolic rate comes to zero.

"When this happens, the physical structure of the nervous system comes to a state where it knows no action. . . . It remains lively, yet without activity. This is that state where there is no decay. . . . Physical decay comes through activity. Cessation of activity results in cessation of the decaying process. . . .

"The field of activity means the field of change, means the field of death, to be permeated, to be supported, to go hand in hand with that which never changes: imperishable, absolute Being [pure consciousness], eternal silence."

This lecture over thirty years ago changed the life of a young student who heard Maharishi's words. The student was Robert Keith Wallace, and after hearing Maharishi and learning the Transcendental Meditation technique, he decided to go into the field of physiology and base his doctoral research on transcendental consciousness and subsequent research on its effects on the aging process.[1]

His dissertation was entitled "The Physiological Effects of Transcendental Meditation: A Proposed Fourth Major State of Consciousness." It earned him his Ph.D. at the University of California at Los Angeles in 1970. His findings were also published in *Science* and *Scientific American*. These articles attracted the attention of the scientific community—which proceeded to replicate Dr. Wallace's studies and corroborate his findings.

Dr. Wallace went on to conduct further groundbreaking research on the TM technique and the physiology of higher states of consciousness. He has written two books, *The Neurophysiology of Enlightenment* and *The Physiology of Consciousness*,[2] and has published many articles in leading scientific journals. He was the founding president of Maharishi University of Management (known as Maharishi International University from 1971–1995) in Fairfield, Iowa and is currently executive vice president, trustee, and chairman of the Department of Physiological and Biological Sciences.

Dr. Wallace has been joined in his research by colleagues all over the world. Studies on the Transcendental Meditation technique now number over 500, conducted in 200 independent universities and research institutions in 30 countries around the world. Studies have been published in dozens of scientific journals.

---

[1] Dr. Wallace tells this story in chapter eight of his book *The Physiology of Consciousness*, published in 1993 by Maharishi International University Press (now Maharishi University of Management Press).

[2] Dr. Wallace's books are available from Maharishi University of Management Press, Press Distribution DB 1155, Fairfield, Iowa 52557.

This chapter will give only a brief overview of the research that has been conducted to date. But for those readers who want to know more, the studies related to the TM technique have been compiled into six volumes entitled *Scientific Research on Maharishi's Transcendental Meditation and TM-Sidhi Program: Collected Papers*, Volumes 1-6 (4,400 pages). These volumes are available from Maharishi University of Management Press, Press Distribution DB 1155, Fairfield, Iowa 52557.

What the Studies Found

The first studies examined what actually happened during the practice of the Transcendental Meditation technique. They showed that oxygen consumption and metabolic rate markedly decreased, indicating a deep state of physiological rest. Breath rate slowed, indicating a more relaxed and rested state of the nervous system. Basal skin resistance, which decreases during times of stress or anxiety, was shown to increase significantly during the practice. Lactate in the blood, also associated with anxiety, decreased. Brain wave patterns were different from those seen in the three well-known states of consciousness—waking, dreaming and sleeping—and indicated heightened inner alertness as well as greater orderliness in brain functioning.

Scientists quickly went on to examine the effects of the TM technique on the subjects' lives, after the actual practice of the technique. What they found was that the TM technique increased perceptual ability, improved reaction time and stabilized the functioning of the nervous system. Meditators recovered from stress more quickly than non-meditators, performed better on complex perceptual motor tests, and learned more quickly. Research also showed improved psychological health in meditators, and an overall development of personality. And there was a marked decrease in the use of both prescribed and non-prescribed drugs.

Excited by the findings, researchers started asking questions. If the Transcendental Meditation technique had profound effects on the physiology during the practice of the technique, and profound

135

effects on subjects' lives after the practice, what were the long-term implications for health? Would it affect one's relationships and family life? Could it be applied in the work environment? Could it be taught in prisons? Were there benefits for students? The military? The government? Would it affect the quality of life for society as a whole?

All of these questions have been asked—and answered by the accumulated body of research on the TM technique.

In the field of health, studies found improved mental and physical health, decreased incidence of disease, reduced need for medical care, younger biological age and extension of life span.

In the area of social behavior, studies found improved self-concept and confidence, improved interpersonal relationships and greater ability to appreciate life and enjoy positive emotions.

In the workplace, meditators showed decreased stress, greater productivity, improved job satisfaction and job performance, and more positive health habits. The number of days lost to sickness and absenteeism dropped dramatically. Studies that examined companies with a majority of employees practicing the technique found that it also improved the bottom line.

When prisoners learned how to meditate, negative traits such as aggression and pathological symptoms were reduced, and in one study prisoners advanced as much in self-development over a one-year period as non-meditating college students typically do in four years. Moreover, recidivism, the tendency of former inmates to return to prison, was sharply reduced.

Students who learned the Transcendental Meditation technique showed greater cognitive development and academic achievement than those who did not learn the technique. They also showed a higher level of principled moral reasoning.

Military commanders who started the TM technique gave powerful testimonials of their experience and recommended that it be applied within the armed forces. Elected officials also started the technique, and encouraged their legislatures to pass resolutions endorsing the practice.

Those who started the Transcendental Meditation technique were enthusiastic, and the scientific studies verified why. Wherever researchers looked, they discovered results that translated into real benefits for everyday life. But the full implications of the TM technique for society as a whole were yet to be realized.

The Maharishi Effect[3]

In the early 1960s Maharishi predicted that if 1% of the world's population practiced the Transcendental Meditation technique, there would be no more war. The peaceful influence of those practicing the technique would radiate throughout the environment and make violence and negative tendencies impossible.

At the time there were not many meditators to test his hypothesis, even on a localized level. But by the mid-1970s, 250,000 people had started the TM technique in the United States alone, and many small cities and towns had 1% of their populations practicing the technique.[4]

Here was a new area of research, and scientists went to work. They started with four "1% cities," and looked closely at their quality of life as measured by crime statistics, accident rates and the number of hospital admissions. The first thing they found was that crime rate did indeed decrease in the 1% cities, when compared to closely matched control cities.

The four cities were expanded to include eleven, then forty-eight, then hundreds of cities in the United States. The results were always the same—a statistically significant decrease in crime resulting from the practice of the TM technique.

---

[3] The discussion of the Maharishi Effect in chapter seven of Robert Roth's excellent book *Maharishi Mahesh Yogi's Transcendental Meditation* (Donald I. Fine, New York, 1994) was an invaluable resource in developing this section.

[4] There are now millions of people practicing the Transcendental Meditation technique worldwide.

This effect, demonstrated so many times, is now called the "Maharishi Effect" in honor of Maharishi. Subsequent research showed that the Maharishi Effect can be intensified and accelerated by the practice of an advanced program of the Transcendental Meditation technique, called the TM-Sidhi program (which includes Yogic Flying). When a group of people practice the TM-Sidhi program together in one place, then the square root of 1% of the population is sufficient to reduce violent tendencies in the environment and create an atmosphere of harmony and positivity.

This intensified Maharishi Effect has been used to calm violence in trouble spots throughout the world, including the Middle East, Central America, South Africa and Southeast Asia. The latest demonstration of this effect took place in Washington, D.C., during one of the hottest and potentially most violent periods the city has ever known. During June and July of 1993, when temperatures soared well over 100 degrees and violent crime was expected to rise accordingly, several thousand experts in the Transcendental Meditation and TM-Sidhi programs assembled to meditate and create a positive "cooling" influence in the environment.[5] As predicted in advance and verified by rigorous statistical analysis, violent crime decreased during those two months compared to expected levels—about 20% by the end of July. Unfortunately, this trend was reversed after the group dispersed and social stress again began to rise.

World peace has been the hope and dream of farsighted leaders throughout the ages. What Maharishi has contributed to this aspiration is the technology to make it a reality. "For the forest to be green, every tree must be green," he has explained. "The individual is the basic unit of world peace. For the world to be at peace, every individual has to be at peace." The Transcendental Meditation technique and its advanced programs are a proven technology to create peace in the individual and society as a whole.

---

[5] The size of the group increased gradually from 800 in June to 4,000 during the last two weeks of July.

Think Big

World peace is health on a global level. And the Transcendental Meditation technique is just one of many Maharishi Ayur-Veda approaches that improve health. Other therapies have been brought to light more recently than the TM technique, and have not, as yet, been researched as thoroughly, but the early studies are promising. For example, the research on Maharishi Ayur-Veda herbal formulas and free radicals has profound implications for the control of disease in its earliest stages.[6] And the simple procedures of seasonal rejuvenation create broad-ranging effects that translate into better health on every level of the mind and body.

Doctors like myself get excited about the research on Maharishi Ayur-Veda therapies because it gives us a vision of possibilities. When I hear debates about how to reform health care in this country, I know that the solution to the health care crisis is at hand. When I see the delicate diplomacy required to keep the world's hot spots under control, I know that the solution to world peace is at hand. When I hear about other problems—in the family, in the workplace, in the economy, in the environment—I know that the Maharishi Ayur-Veda tradition provides a solution.

The Maharishi Ayur-Veda system of health care provides complete knowledge. When this knowledge is applied in its completeness in all parts of the world, we will have transformed the quality of life as we know it on earth.

Heaven on earth begins at home. Through Maharishi Ayur-Veda health care I have already transformed my own life and the lives of many of my patients. I invite you, too, to make your own dreams a reality. There is no time like the present!

---

[6] See chapter seven for a description of free radicals.

Summary

An accumulated body of research on the Transcendental Meditation technique and other Maharishi Ayur-Veda approaches shows profound benefits for health and every other area of life. With the complete application of Maharishi Ayur-Veda knowledge we can create world peace and a heavenly quality of life on earth.

Scientific Research

The following section contains a sampling of the more than 500 scientific research studies on Maharishi Ayur-Veda health care, including studies on the Transcendental Meditation technique (starting on page 142), Maharishi Ayur-Veda herbal formulas (page 167), the Maharishi Rejuvenation program (page 170), and the Maharishi Ayur-Veda system as a whole (page 176).

For more information on the Transcendental Meditation technique see chapter eight.

For more information on Maharishi Ayur-Veda herbal formulas see chapters seven and ten.

For more information on the Maharishi Rejuvenation program see chapter twelve.

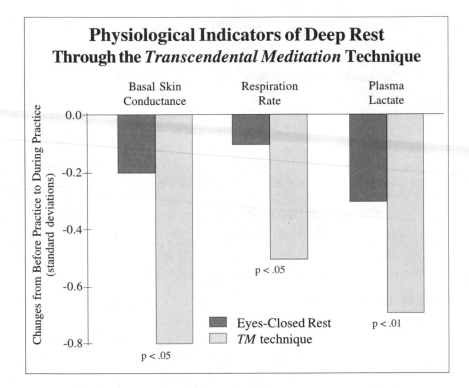

Physiological Indicators of Deep Rest
Through the *Transcendental Meditation* Technique

A meta-analysis (the scientific procedure used for drawing objective conclusions from large bodies of research) found that the Transcendental Meditation technique produced a significant decrease in basal skin conductance compared to eyes-closed rest, indicating profound relaxation in the subjects. Relaxation and deep rest were also indicated by greater decreases in respiration rates and plasma lactate levels compared to ordinary rest.

These physiological changes occur spontaneously as the mind effortlessly settles to the state of restful alertness, pure consciousness, during the practice of the TM technique. Other published studies have demonstrated increased EEG coherence, increased blood flow to the brain, increased muscle relaxation, and decreased stress hormone (plasma cortisol).

References:
1. *American Psychologist* 42 (1987): 879–881.
2. *Science* 167 (1970): 1751–1754.
3. *American Journal of Physiology* 221 (1971): 795–799.

Dr. Reddy's Comments:

More rest is every physician's primary recommendation, because rest gives the body the best chance to heal itself quickly and efficiently. As research shows, the Transcendental Meditation technique gives the entire physiology a unique quality of very deep and rejuvenating rest.

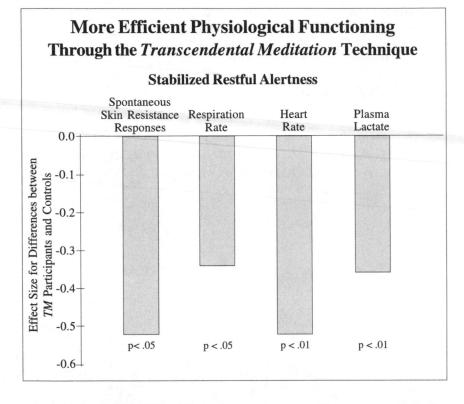

A meta-analysis of published research studies comparing the Transcendental Meditation technique to eyes-closed rest found that those practicing the TM technique have significantly lower baseline levels of spontaneous skin resistance responses, respiration rate, heart rate, and plasma lactate prior to meditation than do comparison subjects prior to rest.

Lower levels of spontaneous skin resistance responses indicate more stability in the autonomic nervous system. Lower respiration and heart rates indicate that the nervous system is less excited and functioning more efficiently. Lower plasma lactate likewise suggests profound relaxation, since high concentrations of lactate have been associated with high anxiety and high blood pressure.

Coupled with extensive research showing that the TM technique increases mental clarity, these findings indicate that the unique state of restful alertness gained during the practice is stabilized outside the practice over time. This more optimal functioning of both mind and body is naturally associated with better mental and physical health (see the following charts).

Reference:
American Psychologist 42 (1987): 879–881.

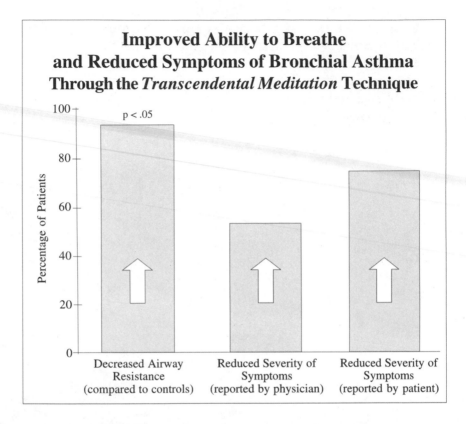

The next day after beginning the practice of the Transcendental Meditation technique, 94% of a group of asthmatic patients showed improvement as determined by the physiological measurement of airway resistance. Their personal physicians reported improvement in 55% of the patients, and 74% reported improvement in themselves.

This study indicates that the TM technique is beneficial for people with bronchial asthma. The severity of bronchial asthma has been consistently correlated with the level of psychosomatic stress of the individual. Because the practice of the TM technique systematically relaxes the nervous system and strengthens its ability to respond to stress, it can be an important treatment for bronchial asthma and other stress-related illnesses.

146

References:
1. *Clinical Research* 21 (1973): 278.
2. *Respiratory Therapy: The Journal of Inhalation Technology* 3 (1973): 79–80.
3. *Respiration* 32 (1975): 74–80.

Dr. Reddy's Comments:

Stress is a major risk factor in all disease, and hampers the recovery process. As this study and others show (see the following charts), the TM technique is a powerful way to combat stress and promote better health.

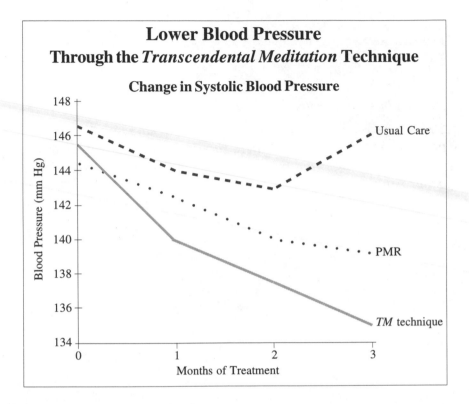

In a clinical experiment with elderly African Americans (mean age 66) dwelling in an inner-city community, the Transcendental Meditation technique was compared with Progressive Muscle Relaxation (a frequently-used method of producing physiological relaxation) and a lifestyle modification education program. Subjects who had moderately elevated blood pressure levels were randomly assigned to the TM technique, PMR, or the education program. Over a three-month interval, systolic and diastolic blood pressure dropped by 10.6 and 5.9 mm Hg, respectively, in the Transcendental Meditation group, 4.0 and 2.1 mm Hg in the PMR group, with virtually no change in the education group. A second random-assignment study with the elderly conducted at Harvard found similar blood pressure changes produced by the practice of the TM technique over three months (11 mm Hg for systolic blood pressure; see page 161).

Hypertension afflicts 43 million Americans and, left uncontrolled, can lead to heart attacks, angina and stroke. As this research indicates, the Transcendental Meditation technique can reduce hypertension significantly.

References:
1. *Hypertension* 26 (1995): 820–827.
2. *Journal of Personality and Social Psychology* 57 (1989): 950–964.
3. *Personality, Elevated Blood Pressure, and Essential Hypertension* (1992): 291.

Dr. Reddy's Comments:

The findings in this study indicate that the TM technique is just as effective in reducing high blood pressure in those with mild hypertension as the usual prescribed medication—and it doesn't cause harmful side effects as medicines often do. In addition, the blood pressure reduction in this study is of a size associated with a 25%–30% decrease in morbidity and mortality due to heart attack and stroke.

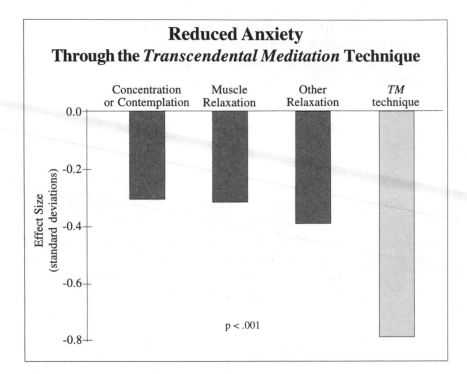

A meta-analysis conducted at Stanford University of all available studies (146 independent outcomes) indicated that the effect of the Transcendental Meditation technique on reducing trait anxiety was much greater than that of concentration and contemplation techniques or forms of physical relaxation, including muscle relaxation. Analysis showed that these positive results could not be attributed to subject expectation, experimenter bias, or research design.

Related studies indicate decreased depression, improvements in post-traumatic stress disorder, more positive self-image, increased integration of self with the social environment, and improved perception of others, in those practicing the TM technique.

References:
1. *Journal of Clinical Psychology* 45 (1989): 957–974.
2. *Journal of Clinical Psychology* 33 (1977): 1076–1078.

Dr. Reddy's Comments:

Anxiety is one of the most common psychological symptoms of stress. Left untreated, it can be a strong contributing factor to many serious physical and mental conditions, including cardiovascular disease, gastrointestinal complaints, asthma, allergies, chronic low-back pain, insomnia and depression. This study indicates that the TM technique is the most effective anxiety-reducing procedure tested to date.

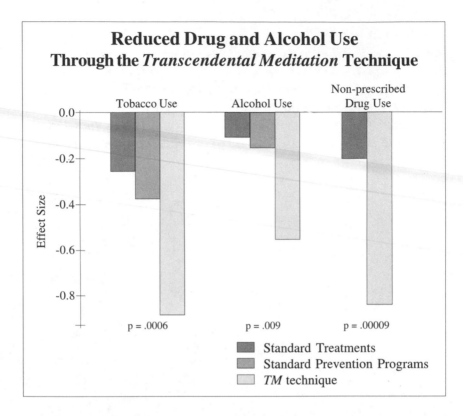

A meta-analysis of 198 independent treatment outcomes found that the Transcendental Meditation technique produced a significantly larger reduction in tobacco, alcohol, and non-prescribed drug use than standard substance abuse treatments (including counseling, pharmacological treatments, relaxation training, and Twelve-Step programs) or standard prevention programs (such as programs to counteract peer-pressure and promote personal development). This meta-analysis controlled for strength of study design and included both heavy and casual users.

Whereas the effects of conventional programs usually decrease sharply within three months, the effects of the Transcendental Meditation technique increased over time, with total abstinence from tobacco, alcohol, and non-prescribed drugs ranging from 51%–89% over an 18–22 month period.

References:
1. *Alcoholism Treatment Quarterly* 11 (1994): 13–87.
2. *International Journal of the Addictions* 26 (1991): 293–325.
3. *Self Recovery: Treating Addictions Using Transcendental Meditation and Maharishi Ayur-Veda.* New York: Haworth Press, 1994.

Dr. Reddy's Comments:

This research corroborates the subjective experience of those practicing the Transcendental Meditation technique—that bad habits such as smoking and drinking tend to fall away naturally over time. It's one of the "side benefits" that often come with regular practice. As meditators experience more inner happiness and satisfaction in their daily activity, they are naturally less attracted to substances such as tobacco, alcohol and drugs.

The costs of substance abuse can be devastating. Alcohol alone is estimated to cause 100,000 deaths in America annually and cigarettes another 400,000—often after long and costly illness. This research shows that the TM technique is more successful in treating substance abuse than standard treatment and prevention programs.

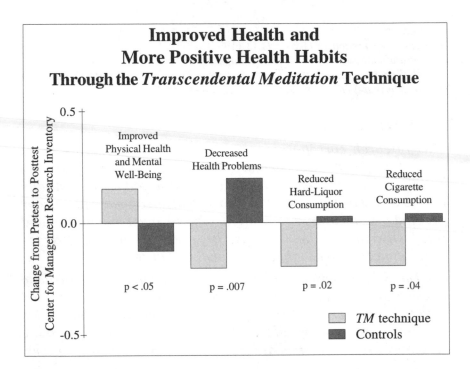

Improved Health and More Positive Health Habits
Through the *Transcendental Meditation* Technique

In two companies that introduced the Transcendental Meditation program, managers and employees who regularly practiced the TM technique improved significantly in overall physical health, mental well-being, and vitality when compared to control subjects with similar jobs in the same companies. Those practicing the technique also reported significant reductions in health problems such as headaches and backaches, a significant reduction in the use of hard liquor and cigarettes, and improved quality of sleep, compared to personnel in control groups.

Related studies indicate that those practicing the TM technique show reduced job worry and tension, decreased desire to change jobs, increased creativity and productivity, improved problem-solving ability, and increased job satisfaction.

Reference:
Anxiety, Stress and Coping: An International Journal 6 (1993): 245–262.

Dr. Reddy's Comments:

Introducing the TM technique into business presents a clear-cut case of a "win-win" situation. The company wins, and the employees win. The company wins by getting better, healthier employees who are more productive. The employees win by improving their health and gaining more fulfillment in their work.

The precipitous rise in health care costs has become a major problem for most companies. This study indicates that the Transcendental Meditation technique has the potential to dramatically control these costs and decrease the number of work days lost to illness. In fact, studies have found reduced health insurance utilization in all categories of disease (see page 157).

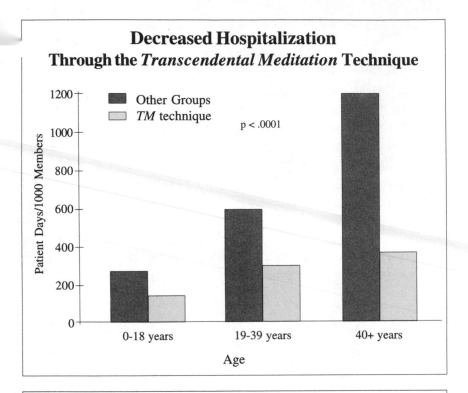

Decreased Hospitalization
Through the *Transcendental Meditation* Technique

■ Other Groups
▢ *TM* technique

p < .0001

Patient Days/1000 Members

1200
1000
800
600
400
200
0

0-18 years   19-39 years   40+ years

Age

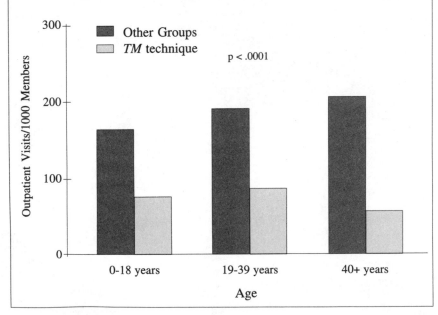

Decreased Doctor Visits
Through the *Transcendental Meditation* Technique

■ Other Groups
▢ *TM* technique

p < .0001

Outpatient Visits/1000 Members

300
200
100
0

0-18 years   19-39 years   40+ years

Age

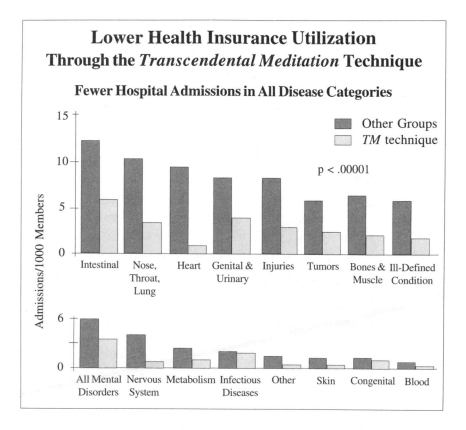

Lower Health Insurance Utilization
Through the *Transcendental Meditation* Technique

Fewer Hospital Admissions in All Disease Categories

A five-year study of health insurance statistics on more than 2,000 people practicing the Transcendental Meditation technique found that they had less than half the doctor visits and hospitalization compared to other groups of comparable age, gender, profession, and insurance terms. The difference between the two groups was greatest in individuals over 40 years of age, indicating that the benefits of practicing the technique are potentially greatest for those facing the greatest risk of disease.

In addition, the study showed that for those practicing the TM technique there were fewer hospital admissions in all disease categories—including 87% less hospitalization for cardiovascular disease, 55% less for cancer, 87% less for diseases of the nervous system, and 73% less for nose, throat and lung problems. The results also showed 76% reduction in major surgery.

These statistics, which document improved health in all age groups and in all categories of disease, indicate that the practice of the TM technique restores balance on a very fundamental level of the physiology. The distinctive state of restful alertness that is gained during the practice allows the immune system and self-repair processes to establish normal, healthy functioning throughout the body, resulting in better general health and the prevention of disease.

This study suggests that the application of the Transcendental Meditation program in the area of health will create substantial savings of financial, medical and human resources. Other research has found substantial reductions in health care costs among those practicing the TM technique.

References:
1. *Psychosomatic Medicine* 49 (1987): 493–507.
2. *American Journal of Health Promotion* 10 (1996): 208–216.

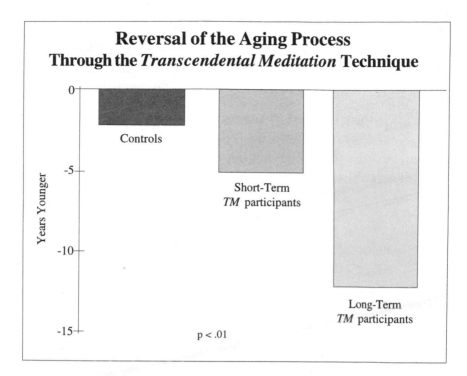

Reversal of the Aging Process
Through the *Transcendental Meditation* Technique

This study examined the effect of the Transcendental Meditation technique on what researchers in the field of aging have called the "biological age" of a person—how old a person is physiologically in contrast to chronologically. As a group, those who had been practicing the Transcendental Meditation technique for more than 5 years were physiologically 12 years younger than their chronological age, as measured by lower blood pressure, better near-point vision, and better auditory discrimination. Short-term TM participants were physiologically 5 years younger than their chronological age. The study statistically controlled for the effects of diet and exercise.

References:
1. *International Journal of Neuroscience* 16 (1982): 53–58.
2. *Journal of Personality and Social Psychology* 57 (1989): 950–964.
3. *Journal of Behavioral Medicine* (1986): 327–334.

Dr. Reddy's Comments:

One of the implications of this research is that the benefits of practicing the TM technique continue to grow over time. We need not lose our youthfulness and vitality as we advance in years. This dispels the myth we take for granted—that with age comes physical deterioration and disease. With the regular practice of the Transcendental Meditation technique and other approaches of Maharishi Ayur-Veda health care, it is possible to live in vibrant, radiant health every day of our life.

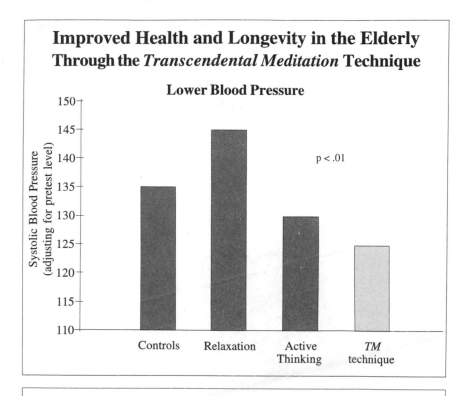

Improved Health and Longevity in the Elderly
Through the *Transcendental Meditation* Technique

Lower Blood Pressure

p < .01

Systolic Blood Pressure (adjusting for pretest level)

Controls   Relaxation   Active Thinking   *TM* technique

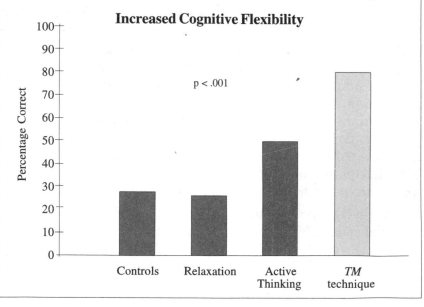

Improved Health and Longevity in the Elderly
Through the *Transcendental Meditation* Technique

Increased Cognitive Flexibility

p < .001

Percentage Correct

Controls   Relaxation   Active Thinking   *TM* technique

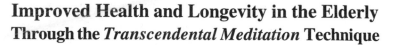

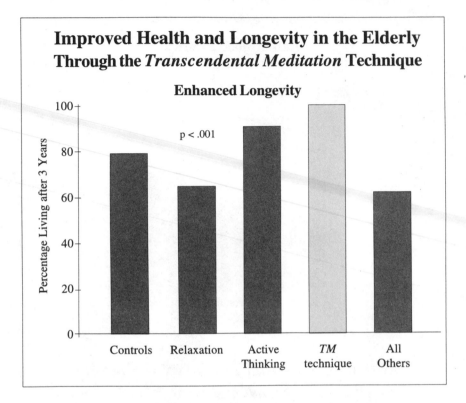

This study randomly assigned residents of homes for the elderly with an average age of 81 years to one of four programs: the Transcendental Meditation program, an active thinking (mindfulness) program, a relaxation program, or a control group with no treatment. Despite similarity among the four groups on pretest measures, expectation, and time spent in practice, the group practicing the TM technique improved most over a three-month period on blood pressure, cognitive flexibility, and other health and cognitive measures. After three years, everyone in the TM group was still alive, in contrast to lower rates of survival for the other groups and a 62% survival rate for the 478 other residents.

A 15-year follow-up study found that average survival time was 22% higher in the TM group compared to the other groups combined.

This experiment shows that declines in health and cognitive functioning can be reversed through the practice of the TM technique even with the advanced elderly, helping them live a longer, happier and more productive life.

References:
1. *Journal of Personality and Social Psychology* 57 (1989): 950–964.
2. *Circulation* 93(3) (1996): Abstracts—A Randomized Controlled Trial of Stress Reduction on Cardiovascular and All-Cause Mortality in the Elderly.

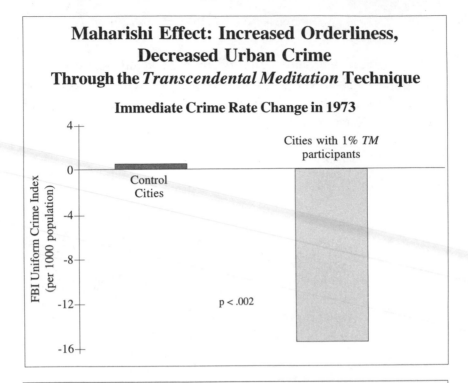

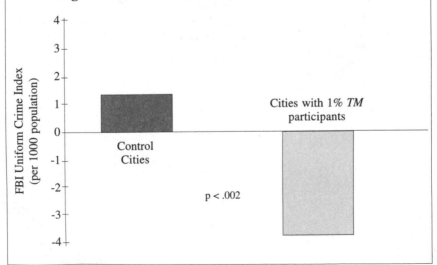

Twenty-four cities in which 1% of the population had learned the Transcendental Meditation technique by 1972 displayed significant decreases in crime rates during the next year (1973) and a decreased crime rate trend during the subsequent five years (1972–1977) compared to 1967–1972. This finding was in contrast to an overall increase in crime in 24 control cities matched for geographic region, population, college population, and crime rate, statistically controlling for a number of other demographic variables.

This effect of a wide-ranging decrease in crime rate cannot be explained by more law-abiding behavior among those practicing the technique or the positive influence they might have on people they directly contact. Instead, this finding indicates that the practice of the TM technique by at least 1% of a population creates an influence of orderliness in collective consciousness from the fundamental level of pure consciousness, which is common to all individuals. This effect of greater coherence in collective consciousness, which is known as the Maharishi Effect (see page 137), results in a reduction of negative trends and an improvement in the quality of life for society as a whole.

Further research in the area of collective consciousness has found that a similar effect is created when a group as small as the square root of 1% of a population collectively practices the TM and advanced TM-Sidhi programs, including Yogic Flying. Published studies have shown: decreased national crime rate; decreases on a national index of homicides, suicides, and motor vehicle fatalities; decreased war intensity and war deaths; more positive, evolutionary statements and actions by heads of state; improvement in national economy; better international relations; increased progress towards peaceful resolution of conflict; and improved quality of city, national and international life, due to increased coherence in collective consciousness created by groups practicing the TM and TM-Sidhi programs.

References:
1. *Journal of Crime and Justice* 4 (1981): 25–45.
2. *The Journal of Mind and Behavior* 8 (1987): 67–104.
3. *The Journal of Mind and Behavior* 9 (1988): 457–486.
4. *Journal of Conflict Resolution* 32 (1988): 776–812.
5. *Social Indicators Research* 22 (1990): 399–418.

Dr. Reddy's Comments:

Crime is a symptom of a diseased society. This study shows that the Transcendental Meditation technique and its advanced programs are a powerful way to reduce crime and improve the health of society as a whole.

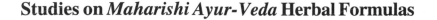

Studies on *Maharishi Ayur-Veda* Herbal Formulas

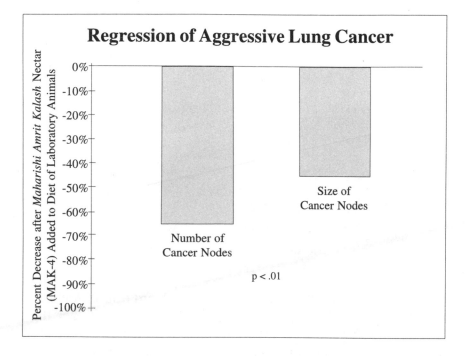

Lewis lung carcinoma is a cancer that aggressively and rapidly spreads to other organs of the body. This kind of cancer is ordinarily the most life-threatening type. In this study, Maharishi Amrit Kalash Nectar (MAK-4) was added to the diet of laboratory animals that already had Lewis lung carcinoma. After 4–5 weeks, the total number of metastatic nodules decreased 65%, while the size of the individual nodules decreased 45%, compared to the control group. (See comments after the following chart.)

Reference:
Nutrition Research 12 (1992): 51–61.

167

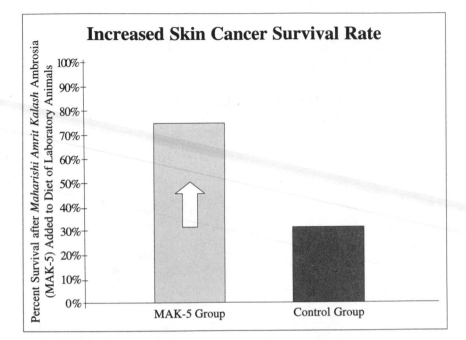

This study examined the effect of Maharishi Amrit Kalash Ambrosia (MAK-5) on laboratory animals with skin tumors. Rather than measure the effect on specific tumors, this study focused on increased survival rate. Animals with chemically-induced skin papillomas were given the formula as a portion (1.5%) of their diet. The survival rate for the animals who were given MAK-5 was 75%, as compared to 31% in the control group. (See comments below.)

Reference:
Pharmacologist 3 (1991): 39 (Abstract).

Dr. Reddy's Comments:

Although this and the previous study apply only to laboratory animals, they give hope to those who are researching cancer treatments for humans. Conventional cancer treatments have grown increasingly sophisticated, but they produce side effects that can be more life-threatening than the disease itself. Moreover, conventional treatments have not been successful in decreasing mortality from the disease or in improving quality of life. Meanwhile, the chances that someone living in the U.S. will die of cancer continue to grow.

Both Maharishi Amrit Kalash formulas are known to be powerful antioxidants (see chapter seven). It is hypothesized that their ability to scavenge free radicals may be responsible for the important results found in these two studies.

Other published studies on these formulas have shown the following results in humans: reduction of the risk of heart disease; improved general health (including improvements in digestion, elimination, sleep, energy, and resistance to illness); decreased worry, depression, and emotional disturbances; and improvement in age-related parameters. Other studies have shown enhanced immune response and reduction of cancer in laboratory animals.

For more on how Maharishi Ayur-Veda herbal formulas work with other approaches of the Maharishi Ayur-Veda system to nourish, balance and strengthen the physiology, see chapter ten.

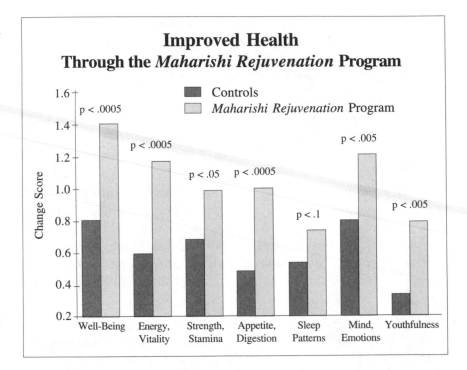

This study compared 142 subjects who participated in a Maharishi Rejuvenation program for one week with 25 control subjects who received only intellectual knowledge of the program and its principles for the same amount of time. Changes in health symptoms were assessed with a health survey questionnaire. Those who received active treatment improved significantly in general well-being, energy and vitality, strength and stamina, appetite and digestive patterns, state of mind and emotions, and youthfulness and rejuvenation. They also reported improvement in previous health conditions. Control subjects did not show the same amount of improvement.

This research indicates that, even after a short period of time, the Maharishi Rejuvenation program simultaneously improves many different areas of health. Other studies have found that this program also improves many aspects of mental health and cognitive performance (see the following charts). These findings support the hypothesis that the Maharishi Rejuvenation program promotes balance in both mind and body on a very fundamental level.

Reference:
The Journal of Social Behavior and Personality 5 (1990): 1–27.

Dr. Reddy's Comments:

More and more doctors are recommending the Maharishi Rejuvenation program on a seasonal basis. According to the tradition of Maharishi Ayur-Veda health care, this seasonal rejuvenation removes accumulated impurities and helps correct imbalances that have built up in the body over time. The treatment is both preventive and therapeutic—it strengthens the body to prevent future disorders as it addresses existing imbalances. This may explain the wide range of benefits that is demonstrated in this and other studies on seasonal rejuvenation.

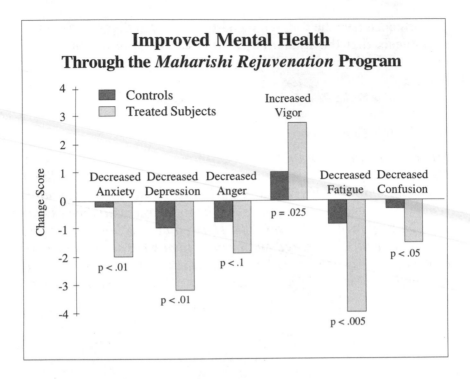

Improved Mental Health Through the *Maharishi Rejuvenation* Program

This study tested 62 subjects before and after participating in a Maharishi Rejuvenation program for one week compared to 71 controls who received only intellectual knowledge of the program for the same amount of time. Changes in mental health were assessed by the Profile of Mood States, a standard psychometric instrument. The results showed statistically significant declines in unhealthy emotional states—anxiety, depression, fatigue, and confusion—and an increase in vigor.

These results indicate the Maharishi Rejuvenation program improves many aspects of the mind and emotions simultaneously. They demonstrate that a physical approach—the purification therapies of seasonal rejuvenation—can have a positive effect on mental health.

Other studies on this program have found increases in intelligence, memory, and alertness (see page 174) and improvements in general health and well-being (see page 170). Taken as a whole, these results indicate that the Maharishi Rejuvenation program promotes better health holistically, by balancing and strengthening both mind and body.

References:
1. Paper presented at the International College of Psychosomatic Medicine, Eighth World Congress, Chicago, Illinois, September 1985: Improvements in Health with the Maharishi Ayurveda Prevention Program.
2. *The Journal of Social Behavior and Personality* 5 (1990): 1–27.

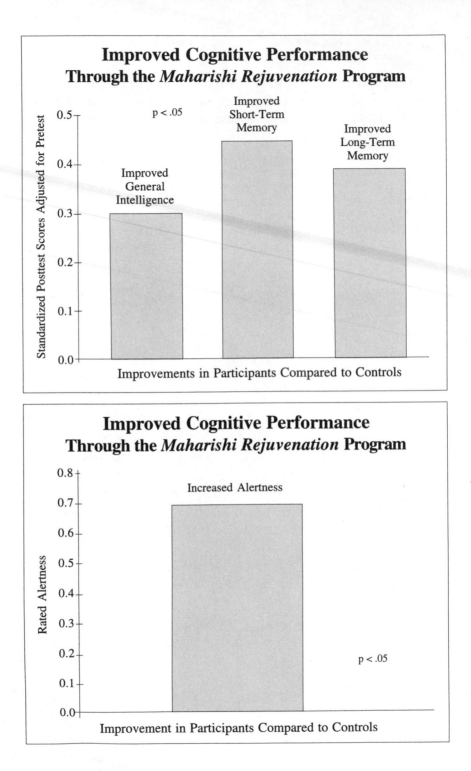

Graduate students who participated in the Maharishi Rejuvenation program improved significantly in comparison to controls on composite measures of general intelligence, short-term memory and long-term memory. Participants also reported significantly greater subjective alertness. Posttest scores were adjusted for pretest levels, and the research also controlled for expectation of benefit, differential motivation, and a variety of other factors.

The Maharishi Rejuvenation program eliminates accumulated impurities and helps to establish balance in the physiology, which results in better physical health (see page 170). Naturally, as physical health improves, mental health improves, and the mind begins to operate more efficiently, which directly improves cognitive performance.

Reference:
Paper presented at the Twenty-Eighth Annual Meeting of the Society of Economic Botany, University of Illinois, Chicago, Illinois, June 1987: Improvements in Memory, Intelligence, Psychomotor Speed Alertness in Normal Subjects from an Ayurvedic Medicinal Herbal-Based Rejuvenal Therapy.

Dr. Reddy's Comments:

This study shows that the Maharishi Rejuvenation program strengthens the physiology to support clear and intelligent thinking. Like the previous study, it demonstrates that a physical approach can produce wide-ranging benefits for the mind. As physiological balance increases, one's thoughts and feelings naturally become more positive, productive and life-supporting.

Maharishi Ayur-Veda health care aims to create total health in mind, body, behavior and environment. The Maharishi Rejuvenation program is only one of many approaches that work holistically to establish balance on all levels at once.

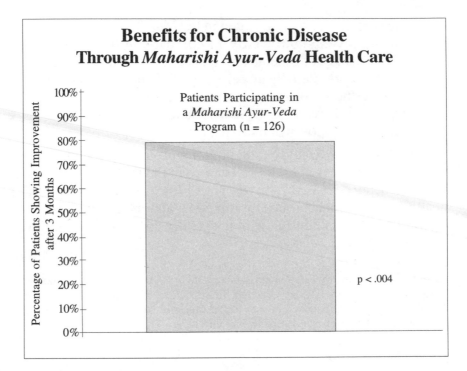

Benefits for Chronic Disease
Through *Maharishi Ayur-Veda* Health Care

Patients Participating in
a *Maharishi Ayur-Veda*
Program (n = 126)

p < .004

(Y-axis: Percentage of Patients Showing Improvement after 3 Months, 0% to 100%)

In cooperation with a health insurance company, a study was conducted at the Maharishi Ayur-Veda Health Center at Laag Soeren, Netherlands, on 126 patients undergoing treatment for chronic diseases. The average duration of illness before treatment was 20 years.

The chronic diseases, which are often resistant to other forms of therapy, included rheumatoid arthritis, bronchial asthma, chronic bronchitis, eczema, psoriasis, hypertension, headaches, chronic sinusitis, chronic constipation, and diabetes mellitus.

The Maharishi Ayur-Veda treatment (individualized for each patient) consisted of a diet program, herbal preparations, and guidelines for daily routine. The patients could also make use of other treatment procedures, including the Maharishi Rejuvenation program and the Transcendental Meditation technique.

Significant improvements were seen in 79% of the patients after three months. Ten patients became completely symptom-free during the period of study. The herbal preparations and other treatment modalities were well tolerated by the patients, and no harmful side effects were noted.

On the basis of this research, it can be seen that within a relatively short time the Maharishi Ayur-Veda approach is able to bring about a substantial improvement in chronic disease, even when it has already existed for many years.

Reference:
Netherlands Magazine of Integrated Science 5 (1989): 586–594.

Dr. Reddy's Comments:

Nearly half of Americans—100 million people—suffer from chronic disease, accounting for nearly three-quarters of the nation's total health care costs. All ages are affected, not just the elderly: one out of every four children has a chronic disease, as do more than one-third of adults age 18–44.

This study offers hope to those suffering from intractable illness. Conventional treatments try to manage the disease, but patients must usually resign themselves to taking prescription medicine for the rest of their lives—medicine that can result in damaging and even debilitating side effects. Maharishi Ayur-Veda health care is effective and generates no harmful side effects. Moreover, it can be combined with conventional treatment without any conflict.

Finally there is a promising solution to the health problems of millions of people—as well as a cost-effective way to address the nation's health care crisis.

Chapter Nineteen

Where to Go for More

Maharishi Ayur-Veda Universities, Colleges and Schools and Maharishi Vedic Universities, Colleges and Schools

The following are partial listings. For other locations, call tcll-free 888-532-7686, or check web site: http://www.Maharishi.org/

In the United States

Albuquerque, New Mexico 505-830-0415
Asbury Park, New Jersey 908-774-9446
Atlanta, Georgia 404-351-9897
Bethesda, Maryland 301-652-7002
Cambridge, Massachusetts 617-876-4581
Chicago, Illinois 312-431-1212
Dallas, Texas 214-821-8686
Honolulu, Hawaii 808-947-2266
Indianapolis, Indiana 317-923-2873
New Haven, Connecticut 203-562-7000
New York, New York 212-645-0202
Omaha, Nebraska 402-345-6656
Pacific Palisades, California 310-459-3522
Palo Alto, California 415-424-8800
Philadelphia, Pennsylvania 215-732-8464
Providence, Rhode Island 401-751-1518
San Diego, California 619-296-6565
Seattle, Washington 206-281-7758
St. Louis, Missouri 314-367-1112
St. Paul, Minnesota 612-225-0872
Tampa, Florida 813-831-7979

In Canada

Compton, Quebec 819-835-5485
Ottawa, Ontario 613-565-2030
Toronto, Ontario 416-964-1725
Vancouver, British Columbia 604-263-2655
Victoria, British Columbia 250-383-9822
Winnipeg, Manitoba 204-957-1434

Short Courses for the Whole Population

1. The *Transcendental Meditation* Program
2. Human Physiology: Expression of Veda and the Vedic Literature (Discovery under Maharishi's Guidance by Tony Nader, M.D., Ph.D.)
3. Good Health through Prevention
4. The *Maharishi Yoga*℠ Program
5. Self-Pulse Reading Course for Prevention
6. Diet, Digestion and Nutrition

These courses are available at all Maharishi Ayur-Veda Universities, Colleges and Schools and Maharishi Vedic Universities, Colleges and Schools (see above). Full descriptions of these courses can be found at web site: http://www.Maharishi.org/

Degree Programs

Bachelor's degree program in Maharishi Vedic Medicine and doctoral degree program in Physiology with specialization in Maharishi Vedic Medicine:

Maharishi University of Management
College of Maharishi Vedic Medicine
Fairfield, IA 52557
515-472-1110
web site: http://www.mum.edu/cmvm/

180

How to Locate a Physician Trained in
Maharishi Ayur-Veda Health Care

Contact your nearest Maharishi Ayur-Veda University, College or School (see above).

Kumuda Reddy, M.D.
1537 Union Street
Schenectady, NY 12309
518-377-0772 (Schenectady)
914-679-5650 (Woodstock)

How to Locate a Teacher of
the *Transcendental Meditation* Technique

Call toll-free 888-LEARN-TM (888-532-7686) or check web site: http://www.tm.org/

Centers Offering
the *Maharishi Rejuvenation* Program

In the United States

Dallas, Texas 214-824-0027
Fairfield, Iowa 800-248-9050
                                       515-472-9580
Lancaster, Massachusetts 508-365-4549
Pacific Palisades, California 310-454-5531
Washington, DC 202-244-2700

In Canada

Compton, Quebec 800-575-5472
                                         819-835-5472
Ottawa, Ontario 613-565-2030

More information is available at web sites:
http://www.Maharishi-medical.com/
http://www.vedic-health.com/

Maharishi Ayur-Veda
Herbal Formulas and Other Products

In the United States

Maharishi Ayur-Veda Products International, Inc.
P.O. Box 49667
Colorado Springs, CO 80949-9667
800-255-8332
719-260-5500
web site: http://www.mapi.com/

In Canada

Maharishi Ayur-Veda Products Canada
P.O. Box 9402
40 Cochrane Road
Compton, Quebec J0B 1L0
800-461-9685
819-835-5485
web site: http://www.all-veda.com/

Recommended Books

Books by Maharishi Mahesh Yogi

Life Supported by Natural Law. Washington, D.C.: Age of

Enlightenment Press, 1986.

Maharishi Forum of Natural Law and National Law for Doctors. India: Age of Enlightenment Publications, 1995.

Maharishi Mahesh Yogi on the Bhagavad-Gita: A New Translation and Commentary, Chapters 1-6. New York: Penguin Books, 1973.

Maharishi Vedic University: Introduction. India: Age of Enlightenment Publications, 1995.

Science of Being and Art of Living. New York: Penguin Books, 1995.

Scientific Research on Maharishi Ayur-Veda Health Care

Scientific Research on Maharishi's Transcendental Meditation and TM-Sidhi Program: Collected Papers, Volumes 1-6, available through Maharishi University of Management Press, Press Distribution DB 1155, Fairfield, Iowa 52557.

Scientific Research on the Maharishi Transcendental Meditation and TM-Sidhi Programs: A Brief Summary of 500 Studies. Fairfield, Iowa: Maharishi University of Management Press, 1996.

Other Books

Nader, Tony, M.D., Ph.D. *Human Physiology: Expression of Veda and the Vedic Literature.* The Netherlands: Maharishi Vedic University Press, 1994.

Denniston, Denise. *The TM Book: How to Enjoy the Rest of Your Life.* Fairfield, Iowa: Fairfield Press, 1986.

Marcus, Jay. *The Crime Vaccine: How to End the Crime Epidemic.* Baton Rouge, Louisiana: Claitor's Publishing Division, Inc., 1996.

O'Connell, David, and Charles N. Alexander. *Self Recovery: Treating Addictions Using Transcendental Meditation and Maharishi Ayur-Veda.* New York: Haworth Press, 1994.

Roth, Robert. *Maharishi Mahesh Yogi's Transcendental Meditation.* New York: Donald I. Fine, 1994.

Sharma, Hari, M.D. *Freedom from Disease: How to Control Free Radicals, a Major Cause of Aging and Disease.* Toronto: Veda Publishing, 1993.

Wallace, R. Keith. *The Neurophysiology of Enlightenment.* Fairfield, Iowa: Maharishi International University Press, 1986.

Wallace, R. Keith. *The Physiology of Consciousness.* Fairfield, Iowa: Maharishi International University Press, 1993.

These books and others are available from Maharishi University of Management Press, Press Distribution DB 1155, Fairfield, Iowa 52557, phone number 800-831-6523. A selection of books is also available from Maharishi Ayur-Veda Products (see information above).

Other Aspects of the *Maharishi Vedic Approach to Health* Program

Maharishi Gandharva Veda[SM] Music

Maharishi Gandharva Veda music is the classical music of the ancient Vedic civilization, the eternal rhythms and melodies of nature. It comes from the same age-old tradition of Vedic knowledge as Maharishi Ayur-Veda health care. Like Ayur-Veda, the knowledge of Gandharva Veda music was restored to its original purity and completeness in this generation by Maharishi Mahesh Yogi. The purpose of this music is to neutralize stress in the atmosphere and create a harmonizing and balancing influence for the individual and society as a whole.

About Gandharva Veda music, Maharishi has explained, "Every level of creation is a frequency. One frequency melts into the other and this is how the process of evolution takes place. The night comes to an end and the dawn begins. At dawn, when the darkness and dullness of the night is over, some inspiring freshness comes and there is a different frequency in the whole atmosphere. At midday, there is another big change in frequency; at evening, a different frequency; at midnight, a different frequency. This cycle of change is perpetual, and because everything is a frequency there is sound at every stage.

"From morning to morning the melody of nature is changing. Gandharva music goes with the time, setting its melodies according to the changing nature. It sets forth those very natural melodies which match with the process of evolution. It provides a powerful harmonizing influence in the whole atmosphere to balance imbalances in nature.

"Gandharva music is the eternal melody of nature spontaneously sung in all levels of creation, from the most minute to the huge, enormous, ever-expanding universe. Gandharva Veda music creates a powerful melody from morning to morning, neutralizing the negative trends and tendencies born of the violation of natural law by the whole population of the world."

Maharishi Gandharva Veda music is available for all 24 hours of the day and night, on audiotape, videotape and compact disk. More information and samples of music can be heard at web site: http://www.Maharishi.org/

For more information on Maharishi Gandharva Veda Music® products:

In the United States

Maharishi Ayur-Veda Products International, Inc.
P.O. Box 49667
Colorado Springs, CO 80949-9667
800-255-8332
719-260-5500
web site: http://www.mapi.com/

In Canada

Maharishi Ayur-Veda Products Canada
P.O. Box 9402
40 Cochrane Road

Compton, Quebec J0B 1L0
800-461-9685
819-835-5485
web site: http://www.all-veda.com/

The *Maharishi Jyotish* and *Maharishi Yagya*^{SM} Programs

The Maharishi Jyotish program—the Vedic science of prediction—is another aspect of the Maharishi Vedic Approach to Health. This knowledge has been applied from time immemorial to help foresee dangers that have not yet come.

Our immediate environment is our home, our neighborhood, our city, country, continent and planet. Our extended environment is the universe around us—other planets, the sun, stars and distant galaxies. The Maharishi Jyotish program deals with this distant environment. Through a Maharishi Jyotish consultation we can identify influences coming to us from our cosmic environment and take proper precautions to avert any negative effect.

The human physiology is part of the cosmic physiology. Every rhythm of the universe naturally has an effect on the individual and vice versa. From the Maharishi Jyotish tradition we have the knowledge of how we interact with our cosmic counterparts.

Maharishi Jyotish knowledge becomes complete with the Maharishi Yagya program. A Maharishi Yagya performance is a precise action based on ancient Vedic wisdom and tradition that restores balance in the functioning of natural law. A Maharishi Jyotish consultation alerts you to a problem, but does not solve it. Maharishi Yagya procedures generate positive influences that restore the synchrony between individual rhythms and the rhythms of the cosmos.

As part of a Maharishi Jyotish consultation, you receive recommendations for any necessary Maharishi Yagya performances to help avert a danger or to enhance the success of an undertaking. Influences that may favor diseases, accidents, lack of success in business, disharmony in marriage or any other problem can be minimized or avoided. A Maharishi Yagya procedure, performed before the danger arises, helps to neutralize negative influences so they do not reach you, and life remains in accord with natural law. Maharishi Yagya procedures may also be performed to enhance good periods in life and bring greater success, prosperity and happiness.

For more information on the Maharishi Jyotish and Maharishi Yagya programs:

In the United States

California 619-754-5197
Illinois 312-341-9978
Iowa 515-472-5603
Massachusetts 617-864-5835
New Hampshire 603-588-4235

For more information call 800-888-5797, or check web site http://www.Maharishi.org/

In Canada

Ontario 613-744-8580

The *Maharishi Sthapatya Veda* Program

Sthapatya comes from the word *sthapana,* which means "to establish." *Veda* means "knowledge." The Maharishi Sthapatya Veda program provides the knowledge of establishment—how to establish the self in pure consciousness, the source of all life, and how to establish one's environment in accord with all the laws of nature so that one always enjoys nature's support.

Maharishi Sthapatya Veda design is the most ancient and supreme system of country, town, village, and home planning in accord with natural law—connecting individual life with cosmic life, individual intelligence with cosmic intelligence, and creating ideal living conditions on earth where everyone will feel, "I am living in heaven."

Maharishi Mahesh Yogi has commented, "Because the individual is cosmic, everything about individual life should be in full harmony with cosmic life. Maharishi Sthapatya Veda design gives dimensions, formulas, and orientations to the buildings that will provide cosmic harmony and support to the individual for his peace, prosperity, and good health—daily life in accord with natural law, daily life in the evolutionary direction."

In response to the urgent worldwide need for people to have ideal working and living environments, Maharishi Global Construction, L.L.C. was established to offer consulting services in Maharishi Sthapatya Veda® design principles to architects, designers and builders. Maharishi Global Construction is currently building 435 Maharishi Vedic Centers, one in each Congressional district throughout the United States, as models of architecture in accord with natural law. These buildings will house all of Maharishi's programs for the development of consciousness and the creation of perfect health, including the treatment and cure of chronic disease. The company is also building 50 in-residence Maharishi Vedic Medical Centers, one in each state, for the treatment of chronic disease through the Maharishi Vedic Approach to Health.

For more information on Maharishi Sthapatya Veda design:

In the United States and Canada

Maharishi Global Construction, L.L.C.
500 North Third Street, Suite 110
Fairfield, IA 52556
515-472-9605
web site: http://www.mgc-vastu.com/

Summary

The Maharishi Ayur-Veda tradition offers many branches of knowledge that address all areas of life. Resources for more information range from courses, books and tapes to web sites on the Internet.

Index

About the Authors

Kumuda Reddy, M.D.

Kumuda Reddy, M.D. has been practicing medicine for twenty years. She completed her residency and fellowship in anesthesiology at Mt. Sinai Hospital, New York.

Dr. Reddy is a former faculty member and anesthesiologist at Albany Medical College. She is currently an adjunct faculty member and practices Maharishi Ayur-Veda health care with conventional medicine in Schenectady, New York. In addition to writing and lecturing extensively on the Maharishi Ayur-Veda approach, Dr. Reddy writes books for children based on the traditional stories of India.

Dr. Reddy lives in Niskayuna, New York with her husband Janardhan, a practicing urologist, and her three children: Sundeep, Suma and Hima.

Stan Kendz

Stan Kendz is founding director of HAPPE Programs, Inc. He is a published author who develops and gives seminars which provide practical solutions to everyday problems. He has a bachelor's degree in biology and a master's of science degree in instructional design. Stan has also been a consultant to high-tech and Fortune 20 companies.

Stan is interested in bringing practical solutions into the field of government and politics, and has run for state offices as a Natural Law Party candidate in 1994 and 1996.

Stan lives in Rochester, New York with his wife Marion Joy and his two children, Matthew and Katherine.

Timeless Stories for Children and Their Parents

Stories written by Dr. Kumuda Reddy and John Emory Pruitt:

The Indigo Jackal
The Monkey and the Crocodile
The Lion and the Hare
The Wish That Came True
The Small Birds and the Great Ocean
The Female Mouse
The Hares and the Elephants
The True Treasure

It is the essential need of our time to help children grow in health and happiness, and to stem the rising crime and violence which plague our society. These traditional stories are full of fun, uplifting values and practical wisdom for everyday life.

Each story is told in a 32-page full-color picture-book format and is available through Samhita Enterprises, Inc.

To contact the authors or for advance notification about other books on Maharishi Ayur-Veda health care:

Samhita Enterprises, Inc.
183 Saint Paul Street
Rochester, New York 14604
1-800-784-2773
E-mail: foreverhealthy@samhita.com
web site: http://samhita.com/forever_healthy